counseling
stutterers

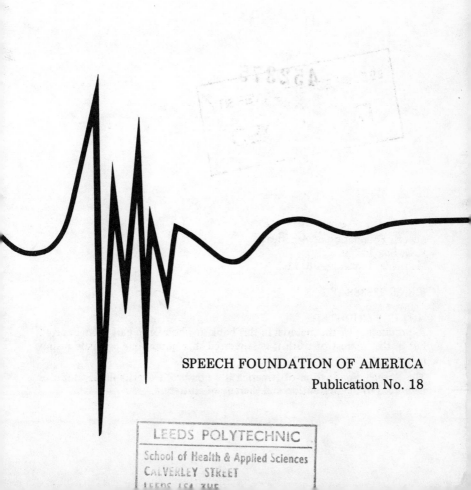

SPEECH FOUNDATION OF AMERICA

Publication No. 18

Speech Foundation of America
P. O. Box 11749
Memphis, Tennessee 38111

ISBN 0-933388-18-7

The Speech Foundation of America is a non-profit charitable organization
dedicated to the prevention and therapy of stuttering.

To the Clinician

This book has been written to give clinicians a better understanding of the counseling aspect of therapy and to provide ways in which it can be used most effectively.

A group of leading authorities in the field of stuttering met for a week-long conference to discuss the role of counseling in the therapy process. They present their ideas in this publication.

Counseling is an important phase of the total therapy process in whatever system of treatment used. Clinical effectiveness should be enhanced by careful consideration of the goals and processes described by these authors.

Jane Fraser Gruss
President

Speech Foundation of America

Conference Participants

Stanley Ainsworth, Ph.D., Chairman

Alumni Foundation Distinguished Professor Emeritus of Speech Correction, University of Georgia. Past President and Executive Vice-President, American Speech-Language-Hearing Association.

Eugene B. Cooper, Ed. D.

Professor and Chairman, Communicative Disorders, University of Alabama. Editorial Board, *Journal of Fluency Disorders*. Editorial consultant, *Journal of Speech and Hearing Disorders*.

Malcolm Fraser

Director, Speech Foundation of America.

Hugo H. Gregory, Ph.D.

Professor and Head, Speech and Language Pathology, Department of Communicative Disorders, Northwestern University. Editorial Board, *Journal of Fluency Disorders*.

Jane Fraser Gruss, Editor

President, Speech Foundation of America.

William H. Perkins, Ph.D.

Professor, Communication Arts and Science, Director, Intensive Therapy Program for Stuttering, University of Southern California. Editor, *Journal of Speech and Hearing Disorders*.

Conference Participants

Joseph G. Sheehan, Ph.D.

> Professor of Psychology, Director, Psychology Speech Clinic, University of California, Los Angeles (UCLA). Editorial Consultant, *Journal of Speech and Hearing Disorders, Journal of Communication Disorders.*

C. Woodruff Starkweather, Ph.D.

> Chairman, Speech Sciences Division, Temple University, Philadelphia. Editorial Board, *Journal of Fluency Disorders.*

Charles Van Riper, Ph.D.

> Distinguished Professor Emeritus and formerly Head, Department of Speech Pathology and Audiology, Western Michigan University. Honors of the American Speech-Language-Hearing Association. Author, *The Nature of Stuttering.*

Dean E. Williams, Ph.D.

> Professor, Speech Pathology and Audiology, University of Iowa. Fellow and formerly Councilor, American Speech-Language-Hearing Association. Editorial Board, *Journal of Communication Disorders.*

Contents

chapter one

The Clinician's Attitudes

Hugo H. Gregory, Ph.D.

The analysis and modification of stutterers' attitudes, and also parents' attitudes when working with children, have been discussed in the literature on stuttering for many years. More recently, the relationship between the client's and clinician's attitude as interacting variables in therapy has received increased emphasis. Consequently, it appears <u>important for clinicians working with stutterers to have a greater awareness of the way in which their thoughts and feelings influence what they do in therapy.</u>

The Clinician's Point of View

At any one time, we are the products of our training and professional experience. When we read a book on stuttering we digest and integrate new information. Every child and adult, including parents with whom we work, probably teaches us something new. Furthermore, when we discuss a client with another clinician, some aspect of the other clinician's perspective usually helps us in understanding our client better. In other words, we are clinicians in the process of change. **A cardinal attitude** we must have as clinicians is to modify our ideas as we give rational attention to new developments and new experiences. We should accept the professional challenge to learn new procedures and to evaluate the results we get when we modify therapy or parent counseling. Beyond this, we can generate new procedures for evaluation and treatment.

Clinicians' Attitudes and the Client-Clinician Relationship

Clinicians' points of view about the nature of stuttering will influence their attitudes about the appropriate relationship between clinician and client. As we know, some writers on stuttering therapy are more specific than others about procedures for modifying the stutterer's attitudes and in discussing the dynamics of the client-clinician relationship. Thus, they also give more consideration to dimensions of the clinician's attitudes. What follows in this chapter is a discussion of clinicians' attitudes based on my experience as a clinician and a teacher.

Understanding the unique feelings and beliefs of the stutterer or parent. One of the characteristics of a therapeutic relationship, often without parallel in a client's experience, is that the clinician enters the relationship with the attitude that each person with a stuttering problem has unique feelings and beliefs and that a situation should be established in which these attitudes are understood as well as possible. In helping my students think about the therapeutic atmosphere that is conducive to the clinician's coming to understand the client better, I suggest that they ask themselves what kind of a person they prefer. Do they like a person who is genuinely interested in them, who takes time to listen, who seems to want to know them better or do they like a person who wants to impart information, to explain circumstances to them? We usually agree that we know more of the givers of information. It may be that giving information expresses dominance and giving direction is related to manipulation and control. Whereas we may view listening and attempting to understand as being indecisive and uncertain. For whatever reason, many student clinicians and professional speech-language pathologists seem to find it easier to be a provider of information and direction.

In my experience, there are three reasons why it is preferable to attempt to understand the client before we give information and make recommendations: (1) Most clients appreciate the interest we show. It is rare that someone has really tried to understand what they have experienced and their perception of it. However, the most important point here is that we should relate the information we give and therapy goals to the person's **unique experience.** (2) What we do early in therapy establishes some of the basic conditions of therapy. If the clinician becomes too directive at the beginning of therapy, the client's main perception of the relationship could be that it is to be one of student and teacher. In this case, we are less likely to get to know some important attitudes of the client. It appears easier to move from being more permissive and understanding to more educational and directive as it is appropriate, than vice versa. (3) one additional reason for the clinician to have this attitude of sincerely wanting to understand is that the process of talking, attempting to describe and explain, will initiate in the client a process of self-evaluation and reorganization of thinking, thus opening the way for that person to receive new information and direction. Thereafter, when the clinician counsels, suggestions can be related to ideas and experiences previously shared by the client. Furthermore, the clinician's accepting and understanding attitude serves as a model for clients' self-acceptance of their present attitudes and behaviors.

In counseling an adult stutterer, the clinician tries to understand how the person feels about his problem, what he thinks caused it, what he has done previously to help himself, and the like. In counseling with parents, we ask them to tell us how they came to be concerned about the child's speech, their observations, their reactions, etc. We listen, ask for clarification and further information. We reward the stutterer or the parents for sharing these perceptions and feelings with us. We are taking a client-centered approach; our previous training and experience help in understanding the general nature of stuttering problems, but we recognize the individuality of their present needs.

To those clinicians who have had only a little experience thus far with stuttering therapy, I should like to mention that earlier in my clinical experience I seemed to have considerable need to impress clients with how much I knew. I want to emphasize here that I do not believe I have ever had clients leave therapy when I was making an honest attempt to understand them as persons with problems.

These statements about counseling in the early stages of therapy emphasize the importance of establishing from the beginning a certain kind of relationship between the clinician and the client. One of the most challenging aspects of being in a helping profession is the necessity to create a positive therapeutic environment for clients with differing cultural, educational, and personal backgrounds. The most successful approach is to show clients, by what you say, that your attitude toward them is one of openness to their unique concerns and experience. Knowing this has always made me more comfortable in counseling because I have not felt that I had to immediately be "the big expert" about each client's problem, and more importantly clients have told me they appreciated it.

Other attitudes of the clinician—being empathic, supportive, and genuine. We have been discussing that time must be given to making a sincere effort to understand the clients' beliefs and feelings as they are verbalized. The clinician expresses this through verbal responses designated as warm, interested, accepting, etc. These verbal responses are expressions of affect. They communicate to clients in a specific way that you are sharing their feelings.

In responding empathically, the clinician is identifying as best he can with the feelings or affective reactions the client is experiencing and communicating this understanding to the client. The clinician presumably recalls some past experience similar to the client's and to some degree re-experiences the event by using self-verbalized cues to evoke the feeling. In other words, if clinicians have experienced sensitivity about some attribute of their own behavior they can identify with the stutterer's sensitivity about speech fluency. If you have experienced the feeling of seeing a child in your family seem frustrated when attempting to do a task and you didn't know for certain what to do, you can perhaps re-experience some of the feeling a mother has when she sees her child "beginning to stutter." In the case of the latter, when the clinician expresses some degree of understanding to the mother, the clinician's empathy is reinforcing to the mother and should increase her willingness to explore her attitudes about her child. The clinician is saying to the mother, "I accept your emotional reactions and you can too! Don't be afraid of your feelings." At the same time, of course, the clincian is seeing that some of his own feelings can be expressed.

A clinician who does not reveal some honest feelings is probably not being genuine. On many occasions I have said to clients, "I have never experienced this particular situation before with other clients and I need to think about it." Even though I am a clinician who still stutters some, or perhaps because I am, I admit that listening to a moderately severe or severe stutterer makes me somewhat uncomfortable. Adult stutterers are especially sensitive to clinicians who appear to be wearing a false face. So, be yourself! Just as the client is an interesting individual to you, you can be an interesting person to the client. However, care should be exercised not to express feelings that could intrude on meeting your client's need or be aimed more toward meeting a need you, the clinician, may have for counseling! For example, as a parent experiencing frustrations with my own children, I have at times felt considerable need when counseling parents to talk about my family situation. While I have considered it appropriate to mention that my wife and I experience somewhat similar difficulties as those discussed with the parents of a stuttering child, I have never allowed the discussion to focus on the specific content of my problems.

You must see your clients' need for support when they come for help, begin to face their problem, explore their attitudes, and seek insight and direction. Recognize that this requires courage and communicate this to them. If you think it desirable for the client to analyze his stuttering pattern, in part by listening on a tape recorder, be aware that this is often difficult, and proceed at an appropriate pace. You may perhaps say: "It is hard to face up to behavior you want so much to avoid."

Providing information and giving directions. We recommend that giving information and direction be de-emphasized during the early stages of the therapeutic relationship. However, from the beginning of therapy every client expects some information and it should be given in a way that will help them clarify their own beliefs and feelings. We have stressed that information and advice or direction will be accepted more readily if clients realize that clinicians have demonstrated a clear interest in understanding their ideas and experiences.

In talking with parents we may give some information about speech development from the babbling stage, to first words, to conversational speech, giving special attention to the concept of normal disfluency. We may talk about factors that precipitate increased disfluency and stuttering. We talk "with" and not "at" them. As information is given the discussion approach encourages an easy exchange of ideas that should be followed. I strongly recommend that all behavior change activity be related to the knowledge we have of the stutterer or the parent as a unique person, and in addition, that we continue to listen carefully throughout therapy to the client's expressions of feelings and thoughts. Clinicians must be flexible, recognizing that their roles change as therapy progresses. At first, as I have suggested, the clinician may be more permissive and understanding, then more directive and supportive, then challenging with an element of confrontation, and finally encouraging independence. These behaviors are timed appropriately depending on the clinician's evaluation of the client's behavior, feelings, and understanding. For example, when stutterers are experiencing new successes in speaking situations the clinician can challenge them to do more.

Clinicians' attitudes toward themselves. We all respond to ourselves as well as to others. When we think about ourselves, we have varying degrees of self-confidence. If we wish our clients to have more realistic attitudes we should have the desire to be more realistic about ourselves. We discussed at length the goal of understanding clients as unique individuals. Likewise, we must attempt to increase our awareness of our uniqueness — our areas of self-confidence and our insecurity.

Joseph Sheehan's comments about clinicians' stuttering equivalents have always been helpful to students. Sheehan observes that nearly everyone has equivalent problems, such as an unusual facial structure, a scar, etc., and he believes that the fascination that stuttering holds for many people is explainable on this basis. From the equivalents of stuttering come an opportunity for understanding by the clinician. Since every therapist builds his therapeutic style around his own personality, this is a feature he can share with the stutterer.*

---

*See Sheehan, J. Role therapy. In Sheehan, J. (ed) Stuttering: research and therapy. New York: Harper and Row, 1970. pp. 282-283.

With reference to working with stutterers, be realistic. If you are reading this book, you are interested in the problem of stuttering, but you could be a speech pathologist who does not wish to include stutterers in your practice. Possibly, you would like to specialize with children and the prevention of stuttering. If you feel insecure at present about working with adult stutterers, then admit this and if motivated to do so, proceed to secure additional training. In any case, be honest about your present knowledge and experience or feelings about the problem of stuttering as compared to other communicative disorders.

Have you developed some self-confidence about your ability to use a problem solving approach to analyze and work with some of your own personal difficulties? For example, have you defined a problem, thought of several possible solutions, chosen one, carried it out, and then evaluated the results? Obviously, this is one of the procedures your client has to utilize in therapy, so you will be more effective if you have used this approach successfully in your own life. Have you monitored your sensitivity to criticism, your need to rationalize about your behavior, or your tendency to project into others an attitude that in reality is an attitude you have toward yourself? Regarding criticism, parents and other clients will sometimes question what you say or recommend. Can you recognize that you may have some emotional response to the point of the criticism or the person's manner of being critical; yet realize that you should attempt to understand and that whatever you accomplish constructively must take this criticism into account. Concerning rationalization, if you recognize and accept in yourself a certain degree of this mechanism of justifying ideas and behavior in a way that seems reasonable to you, you can help your clients have a realistic appreciation of this self-attitude. Furthermore, you can evaluate with more insight and objectivity the way in which you may be justifying a response to a client, e.g., giving an interpretation, in counseling. Finally, an awareness of projection, the tendency to see ourselves in others, should help us to make decisions that are based more properly on the client's needs. To expand our self-awareness, we should participate in self-study programs that help us through interaction with others to have increased insight into our own attitudes and behavior. Being an effective counselor requires a lifetime of self-study.

Referral for psychotherapy. All clinicians working with stutterers should be able to deal with the attitudinal and behavioral characteristics related to the frustrations of stuttering and the concerns of the parent of a child beginning to stutter or a child having a more confirmed problem. However, some stutterers or parents of children who stutter may need broader forms of personal guidance if their insecurity or inadequacy is more pervasive and interferes with their ability to profit from therapy. The speech clinician should recognize that other specialists such as psychologists and social workers may contribute usefully to the understanding of a client's problem and appropriate therapy. In some clinics, this need is recognized at the beginning of therapy by including a psychological consultation in the evaluation procedure. Other clinicians observe adjustment patterns during therapy and refer for consultation and psychotherapy as the need is recognized.

If we establish a situation in which clients are comfortable to communicate, we may become aware of client needs that go beyond our competence. When psychological insecurities and conflicts not so directly related to the speech problem are expressed, we should be calm and understanding. However, we should immediately begin to consider the possibility of a referral. Here are a few signs of the need for psychological referrals that I have experienced recently: An adult stutterer revealed that he was frightened by his feelings of hostility although most people viewed him as passive. A female stutterer reported concern over persistent unhappiness for which there did not appear to be a reason. A parent of a four year old child who was beginning to stutter expressed her bewilderment over the responsibility of caring for her children and use of appropriate discipline. Finally, a mother, counseled about a child stutterer's home environment, revealed that her married life had been unsatisfactory for several years.

My approach is to express confidence in the psychologist, social worker, marriage counselor, etc., to whom a referral is made. Furthermore, I express the idea that we all deserve help from time to time in resolving questions we have about our lives. People who stutter, or their parents, may or may not have other problem areas of concern.

The clients' success. Stuttering is cyclic in occurrence and severity and the clinician must plan to help stutterers and the parents of stuttering children to understand that, in therapy and following formal therapy, provision should be made for coping with degrees of regression. This happens to some extent with other speech problems, but we should realize that transfer and maintenance require substantially more attention and time in stuttering therapy. The clinician who understands this can help the client to have this realistic perspective.

If we are realistic about the time commitment involved, I believe the results of work with stutterers can be quite favorable and rewarding when compared with that of other types of speech problems. Careful and frequent measures of speech in various situations and self-reports of progress help clients realize the results of therapy more objectively. In this way the clinician and the client can be realistic about progress. Sometimes in spite of our best effort to reinforce the client and to maintain motivation, stutterers will not continue their effort and results will suffer. But we will never find a profession in which we will not at times be uncomfortably anxious about our decisions and suffer some guilt feelings. We must ask ourselves whether we are giving sufficient thought to our clients and planning to meet their needs as best we can. Success is probably not as absolute and immediate as we and clients may wish — or that sensational newspaper articles may imply.

Conclusion

Self-study is an active process in which all clinicians should be engaged throughout their professional careers. The resulting insight into our feelings, beliefs, and behavior (and the way in which these three are related) increases our objectivity as we evaluate clients and make decisions about treatment. Our point of view at any one time influences the way we perceive a stutterer's problem. We should remain open to new information and ideas. Stutterers and parents of stuttering children are viewed as unique individuals whom we wish to understand, with a need for empathy, support, direction and reinforcement, and finally, with differing needs as therapy progresses. The more realistic clinicians are about themselves, the more able they are to respond positively and constructively to their clients.

chapter two

Understanding the Process

Eugene B. Cooper, Ph.D.

Introduction

The extent to which speech clinicians have used counseling procedures in their therapy for stutterers has varied markedly during the past three decades. During the nineteen sixties there was a shift away from counseling to an emphasis on behavioral programs. While many clinicians of the 50's held that the development of objective attitudes on the part of stutterers towards their stuttering and themselves would lead to increased fluency, many clinicians of the 60's and 70's focused instead on the reinforcement or punishment of behaviors that would result in an increase in fluency. It was assumed that the clients' stuttering-related attitudes and feelings would no longer be a problem once the disfluent behavior was eliminated. By the middle of the 1970's many clinicians felt that while fluency shaping programs were eliciting fluency in the stutterers treated, counseling was also needed by many of those same stutterers if they were to increase and maintain their fluency.

Too frequently, clients entering a behaviorally-oriented stuttering program believed that their stuttering behavior would be changed for them. They concluded that all they had to do was to follow the programmed instructions and with no mental or physical effort they would allow the reinforcing or punishing contingencies carry them to a lasting fluency. Unfortunately, such is not the case. Research has demonstrated that almost any stimulus made contingent upon disfluencies in clinical situations serves as a "punisher" resulting in increased fluency in that situation. Clinical experience, however, has shown that fluency resulting from such clinical manipulations is temporary unless the stutterer is aware of and emotionally committed to maintaining the behavioral patterns established during the therapy program.

By the end of the 1970's and the beginning of the 1980's, many clinicians were again emphasizing the need for counseling activities in the stuttering therapy process. They felt that counseling procedures could be integrated successfully with behavior modification techniques and would assist the stutterer in adjusting to changes. How clinicians use counseling in stuttering therapy, of course, varies with the clinician's ideas about the cause of stuttering and the goals of stuttering therapy. This chapter begins with a description of three variables which may be assessed to determine the need for including counseling procedures in a stuttering therapy program and concludes with the description of a counseling process with stutterers.

Variables Indicating Need for Counseling

We know that stutterers do not possess characteristic personality traits. As a group they are no different from groups of normally fluent speakers with respect to the presence or absence of psychopathology. We also know that chronic stutterers, like other groups of individuals with observable disabilities, may develop behaviors, feelings, and attitudes which impede therapy. Counseling appears appropriate when the stutterer's progress in therapy is impeded by 1) misperceptions, 2) emotional overlay and 3) a disparity between the way the stutterer thinks and feels about himself and his stuttering.

Misperceptions. Some stutterers have very few misperceptions. They can accurately describe the way they stutter. They see the ramifications of their stuttering clearly and are able to accurately assess the reactions of others to their stuttering. Such stutterers probably need little counseling and can begin immediately to make behavioral changes as directed by the clinicians. Other stutterers are less fortunate. They may not be aware of what they do with their tongue, lips, and jaw during the moment of stuttering. They may think that their stuttering does not interfere with communication when in fact it does. They may think that their speech is so disfluent that every listener is pained by their speech when, in fact, most of their listeners are not even aware of their stuttering. These stutterers will need counseling.

Emotional Overlay. Perceptions which directly affect our self-concept are more charged with emotion than those having little relevance to it. We feel strongly when someone challenges our feelings of self-worth but little or no emotional response when informed of an event with no relevance to our own lives or beliefs. It is difficult to get a child or an adult to work on his speech if he does not feel it is important. It is much easier to get a person to work on his speech if he feels his speech is important and his feelings of self-worth are threatened by his poor speech. In some instances, the stutterer's feelings of hopelessness and defeat based on misperceptions of the stuttering problem may be so strong that he may not even want to enter therapy. Obviously, in such a case, counseling would be necessary. Misperceptions with little or no emotional significance can normally be altered through instruction, whereas misperceptions overlaid with feelings require a counseling relationship.

Disparity Between Thoughts and Feelings. The clinician should consider the lack of harmony between the way an individual thinks and feels about himself. A stutter may **know** he is bright but may not **feel** he is. A stutterer may be **intellectually** aware of the need to modify his speech but may not be **emotionally** committed to doing so. When the disparity between the stutterer's thoughts and feelings is significant, counseling may be necessary to help the stutterer to come to terms with himself.

In view of the three variables noted above, counseling appears appropriate when the stutterer:

1. has significant misperceptions about his stuttering and about the ramifications of his stuttering problem;

2. has feelings about his stuttering or himself that will significantly impede his use of fluency enhancing procedures and his ability to communicate effectively and;

3. experiences significant discrepancies between the way he thinks and feels about his stuttering and himself.

Problems in the three areas noted above will gradually become evident to the stutterer's clinician as the client's stuttering behavior and related attitudes are identified during the evaluation process prior to the initiation of therapy. The stutterer's behavior and attitudinal patterns that may indicate the need for counseling will become even more evident to the clinician as the client begins to make efforts to modify the stuttering behavior. If the clinician finds no problems in the areas noted above, he may assume that counseling is not necessary. In that case, he can proceed with focusing on teaching the stutterer fluency enhancing techniques. Conversely if he finds that problems exist in one or more of the three areas, the clinician may assume that counseling will be needed to obtain long-term fluency.

In a few instances, the stutterer's problems in each of the three areas noted above will be of such a magnitude that the clinician will refer the client for a psychological evaluation to determine if psychotherapy is needed. In most instances, however, he will find that the chronic stutterer, although possessing therapy-impeding feelings, attitudes, and behaviors, will have sufficient intellectual and emotional integrity to benefit from the counseling process. Because the success of counseling is dependent primarily upon the client's ability to participate in the interchange of feelings and ideas between the client and clinician, counseling appears appropriate for those who are 1) in touch with reality, 2) capable of rational thought, and 3) have the potential for initiating and sustaining emotionally significant interpersonal relationships.

The Counseling Process

Counseling has been defined as the mutual exploration and exchange of ideas, attitudes, and feelings between a counselor and a client. In counseling, the clinician encourages clients to explore and to clarify, primarily by thinking out loud: their thoughts, feelings, and attitudes about their problems. Subsequently, based on the client's better self-understanding, the clinician assists the client in making his own decisions about what changes to make.

Obviously, the relationship between the client and the clinician is a critical variable in successful counseling. Terms such as "warm," "personal," "supportive," "nurturing" and "friendly" have been used to describe this relationship. Such terms do not always describe the significant changes in client's feelings about the clinician, the client-clinician relationship, and the activities that typically occur during a successful therapy process. The client may not **always** see the clinician as being "supportive" or "friendly." Many counselors go so far as to suggest that a counseling relationship in which the client always feels totally comfortable may even delay progress. They suggest that client self-evaluation activities (perhaps **the** critical activity in counseling) are stimulated most effectively when the client and clinician, through open and honest interchanges of feelings, attempt to resolve the uncomfortableness brought about by the client's negative feelings toward the clinician and the process. In fact, the counseling process may best be described on the basis of the typical changes that occur in client's feelings as counseling proceeds.

The following description of therapy with stutterers encompassing counseling activities focuses on how the clinician, by being aware of the stutterer's feelings about the clinician and the therapy, can facilitate attitude and behavior changes. The extent to which stutterers will experience the feelings described in the process will vary markedly from stutterer to stutterer. However, we know that the pattern of changes in feelings described below appears to be typical of all helping relationships. The process is described as having four stages which highlight the therapeutic activity and the resulting feelings of the stutterer.

1. Orientation. Counseling begins with the clinician giving the client an idea of the goals and a description of what to expect. The clinician notes how important the client-clinician relationship is and suggests that the relationship will undoubtedly be a topic of many discussions, particularly in the early stages. Also in the initial sessions, the clinician and the client begin the process of cataloguing and defining those behaviors, thoughts, feelings, and attitudes that constitute the stuttering problem.

Clients usually become more positive in their feelings toward the clinician and the process during their first session. This probably happens because the identification and cataloguing of stuttering behaviors and attitudes reduces anxiety. From a vague pervasive problem, stuttering has become more understandable and the stutterer is reassured. Now he can organize his thinking and focus on what to do. In addition, the clinician's description and structuring of the therapy process reassures the stutterer that something can and will be done. These initial positive feelings become more important during the second stage of therapy when the relationship becomes more involved and more stressful and the client becomes less positive.

2. Relationship. The second stage of counseling begins when the clinician and client focus on what to do. The specific aspects of the stuttering problem on which the clinician will focus will depend, of course, on his orientation to stuttering therapy. He may suggest modifying eye or hand movements during moments of disfluency or, if using a structured program, may begin teaching fluency initiating activities such as conversational rate control. Regardless of what specific adjustments are suggested, the stutterer begins to feel pressure to make changes. These pressures naturally result in resistances that may occur even though the client appears to be making efforts to initiate change. For example, the client, finding that it is not so easy to modify the stuttering, may begin to deny the significance of the stuttering. In another instance, the stutterer may begin to intellectualize about the problem rather than to face the real feelings being generated by the pressures for change. In still another instance, the stutterer may simply give up, stating that he is incapable of doing the things being suggested by the clinician.

The nature and strength of the resistance that the client exhibits may give the clinician a clue about how therapy will progress and perhaps, about the client's prognosis. Of course the clinician is interested not just in the client's resistances but also in the client's attitudinal and behavioral patterns that should facilitate change. Thus, the relationship stage of counseling begins with the stutterer beginning to make changes and the clinician observing the client's reactions to his attempts. At this point in therapy, clients typically become less positive toward the clinical process and the clinician. Often they are disappointed when they realize that the clinician can wave no magic wand to create fluency and that they must earn it through a long and arduous process of speech adjustments and self-monitoring.

The effective clinician is one who, understanding the inevitability of client resistances and disappointments at this stage of therapy, encourages the client to express these negative feelings. In fact, the skillful clinician uses these negative feelings to help the development of an open and honest clinical relationship which is necessary if counseling is to succeed. The manner in which a stutterer's attention is drawn to his resistances and negative feelings is critical to the counseling process. The clinician draws the client's attention to the resistances and feelings in such a manner that the stutterer sees the clinician as not being judgmental but as being open, honest, and above all, as having positive regard for the client. To be successful in initiating an open and honest relationship, the clinician's verbalizations must be based on accurate observations; they must be to the point; and they must carry with them the clinician's sense of respect and caring for the client as well as his belief that the client can make positive changes.

When clients understand that their expressions of negativism are accepted, they will express their feelings more openly and will begin to feel more comfortable in the relationship. In such an atmosphere, clients find that they can explore, examine, and discuss their feelings without the fear of being judged or misunderstood. The relationship stage of the counseling process is successfully completed when the client feels free to express both negative and positive feelings openly, to think out loud, to exchange ideas with the clinician, and to engage in self-evaluation without being judged by other people's standards. In such a relationship, the stutterer will not only adopt the clinician's presumably more accurate perceptions of the stuttering problem, but will begin to compare his own reactions to the problem with the clinician's. As the key factor in providing the stutterer with better ways of viewing and valuing his stuttering, himself, and his fluency goals, the clinician may become a "reality check" for the client.

3. Adjustment and Planning. During the adjustment phase of the third stage of therapy, the client begins to correct misperceptions, to place his feelings in proper perspective, and to reduce the disparity between his thoughts and feelings. These changes will occur if the client has come to value positively the clinician's attitudes and feelings. It was noted that in the second stage of therapy, much of the time was spent discussing the client-clinician relationship, and there was an almost even interchange of verbalizations. In the adjustment phase, however, the stutterer does most of the talking and thinking out loud. The clinician simply reflects and clarifies what the client says. When the clinician feels that the client's perception of the problem and himself is relatively accurate, the clinician may begin the planning phase of the third stage of therapy.

In the planning phase, the stutterer and the clinician establish mutually agreed upon goals. The degree to which the clinician takes the lead in identifying these goals will depend on the client's age, his abilities, the behaviors and attitudes to be modified, and the clinician's orientation to stuttering therapy. Obviously, young children will need the clinician's direction. The complexity and severity of the client's pattern of disfluencies, and the extent to which the client's attitudes and feelings may hinder or help change, will also help determine how much responsibility the clinician assumes.

Clinicians favoring fluency shaping programs will suggest fluency goals already established within the therapy program being used. Other clinicians may help the stutterer set his own goals after giving him a chance to explore various options for fluency control. Clinicians favoring a programmed therapy approach generally see the goal-setting phase as a discrete and brief phase of therapy. The clinician describes the program and, when the issues raised in the relationship stage of therapy are resolved, leads the client into the fourth and final stage of therapy. Clinicians who believe that therapy goals should be developed as therapy progresses continue the goal-setting activities initiated in this stage throughout the final stage of therapy. In the adjustment and planning stage of a successful therapy process, a key feature of the client-clinician relationship is the significant increase in the client's positive feelings toward the clinician and the therapy.

4. Application.   The final stage of therapy might be described as being primarily instructional in nature. The assumption is made that the stutterer, having progressed through the initial stages of therapy, sees himself and his problem accurately, has identified his goals and, to achieve those goals, needs only instruction in the application of specific techniques. The specific techniques used to elicit fluency in stutterers will, of course, vary according to the clinician's approach to stuttering therapy. Clinicians may approach fluency control by teaching the stutterer to stutter more fluently by superimposing voluntary behaviors over the involuntary moments of stuttering. Others may focus on altering the stutterer's habitual speech patterns to maintain acceptable fluency in all situations. Both approaches have been found to be effective in eliciting increased fluency.

During the final stage of counseling, the interchange of feelings between the client and clinician stabilizes. Whereas a significant decrease in the stutterer's positive feelings toward the clinician and the therapy is characteristic of the second stage of therapy and a significant increase in positive feelings is characteristic of the third stage, the fourth stage is characterized by a leveling-off trend. In fact, in many instances, as the stutterer prepares himself for the termination of therapy, a gradual decline in his positive feelings is observed. Such a decrease in positive feeling has been interpreted as an indication of the stutterer's healthy withdrawal from dependency on the clinician. A successful therapy process is concluded when the stutterer has gained a better understanding of himself and his problems, has developed strategies for resolving the problem to the extent possible, and thinks and feels that he can maintain his gains without a formalized therapy relationship.

chapter three

The Severe Young Stutterer

Charles Van Riper, Ph.D.

In a long career some of the toughest problems that I have encountered have been those presented by very severe young stutterers, especially those who seem chock full of frustration, fear, shame or other unpleasant feelings. These children hurt badly and they show it. Because they find it hard to talk, it is difficult to establish a good clinical relationship. To them, communication is a very painful experience to be undertaken only when absolutely necessary. Often hostile or withdrawn, these children are very difficult to help until some of that bottled up emotion is vented.

My early attempts to provide some emotional release for these young severe stutterers were the traditional ones: play therapy, simplified verbal counseling, psychodrama, free-smearing techniques and the like. I was not at all impressed with the results I got. While these procedures did enable the children to act out a lot of their conflicts with their parents, siblings or playmates, they did not focus at all on the feelings engendered by the stuttering itself. They could beat up inflated Bozo the Clown enthusiastically but that didn't seem to help them respond to their blockings with any less frustration or struggle. To me, these young stutterers seemed to need some immediate release, some instantaneous way of expressing the feelings that boiled up in them at the moment of stuttering. At first I thought that I could verbalize for them, trying to put into simple words what I thought they were feeling, but it soon became evident that this was not doing the job that needed to be done. The children, shortly after having a very severe moment of stuttering, seemed to be too full of emotion even to hear what I was saying. Moreover, I was doing too much talking and they were doing little or none. Some other way had to be found to help these young severe stutterers ventilate and discharge the unpleasant feelings that arose when they stuttered.

After considerable exploration, I developed some essentially nonverbal techniques that eventually led to the child stutterers' being able to share their feelings with me. And then I found not only a marked though temporary increase in fluency but also a willingness or capacity for modifying their stuttering behaviors, behaviors that earlier had been very resistant to change.

The essence of this approach requires the clinician to mirror **nonverbally** first the overt stuttering behaviors and then the unpleasant feelings that the child experiences when he stutters. Verbal mirroring, usually termed reflecting, has long been used in psychotherapy, the clinician attempting to verbalize in his own words the feelings being expressed by the client, or which underlie what the latter is telling him. With normal speakers, if the therapist's reflection is inaccurate, the client will verbally reject the interpretation but many stutterers, and especially the younger severe ones, find this contradicting difficult to do. Therefore, misunderstandings arise that threaten the relationship. Nonverbal mirroring avoids this hazard to some extent since the clincian's symbolic behavior can be interpreted by the child in various ways. Thus he tends to read into it the interpretation most consonant with his actual feelings.

The targets of this nonverbal mirroring are the same ones that have always been viewed as essential: to reduce and help the stutterers cope with their feelings of helplessness, frustration, anger, fear and shame. Improvement in fluency almost always seems to result when these unpleasant responses are weakened, and when they are decreased, both the stutterer and his clinician find the other work of therapy much easier.

Before we go on to describe the actual procedure of nonverbal mirroring we should make clear that although the emphasis is upon nonverbal interactions between the clinician and the child stutterer, this does not mean that the sessions are completely silent. While the clinician rarely asks a question or insists upon a reply, some brief commentary often occurs and it is always necessary to do some talking to structure the therapeutic tasks.

We have always begun our therapy with any stutterer by first exploring together the problem he presents. With a child, we might begin by saying, "I'm going to help you be able to talk more easily but I've got to learn first exactly what happens when you stutter and I guess you'll have to teach me. The next time you have some trouble saying a word you'll see me having it too. I'm not mocking you; I'm trying to understand what happens." Then when the child does stutter noticeably we (occasionally) stutter right along with him, trying to duplicate what he is doing. Early in the sessions, we do this on the milder blockings and in pantomime only but later we will mirror the hard ones too and aloud. Often we may insert a bit of commentary like this: "No, I didn't do it quite right that time. Forgot to squeeze my lips as tightly as you did. Let me try it again." The major work of the first sessions consists of this mirroring and brief commentary. Sometimes we do it simultaneously with the child; at other times, we echo the stuttering behavior.

Now let us examine the impact of this simple mirroring in terms of its psychodynamics. The child's first reaction is that of surprise; the second, that of suspicion. These soon dissipate as the clinician shows his earnestness and his genuine interest in the stuttering being exhibited. The next reaction is one of relief. The child realizes that here is one adult who is not repelled or appalled by his stuttering. Here is one grown-up who is willing to put into his own mouth the dirty stuff that everyone else rejects and penalizes. And he doesn't seem at all upset or ashamed when he stutters. He's curious about it; he's not afraid to stutter. When these reactions occur, the child no longer feels so terribly alone and helpless. His burden, being shared, is thereby lessened. Perhaps here he has one grown-up he can trust.

In the next phase of this approach the concentration is not primarily on the stuttering behaviors being exhibited but on the feelings that exist concurrently. The clinician introduces this new interaction by saying something like this: "I think I've now pretty well learned what you do when you stutter, and maybe you have too. Now let's see if I can understand how you **feel** at the time you stutter or just before or afterwards. I'll try to act out what I think your feeling is and if I'm wrong, let me know."

Since the symbolic mirroring of feelings occurs spontaneously and in a specific context, it is difficult to describe it here in print. I know that often I have locked my fingers together and vainly tried to pull them apart when I felt that the child was feeling very frustrated at the moment of hard blocking. There were times when I drooped bodily or whimpered when I thought he was feeling helpless. I have banged the walls and the table if he seemed hostile. There were instances when I covered my face as a gesture of shame, others when I assumed the mask of fear. Often, of course, I failed to mirror the actual feelings, having misinterpreted them, but when that occurred, the child usually corrected me. Once, for example, after a young stutterer had experienced a very long, compulsive series of repetitions that seemed to last interminably, I felt that he must have been terribly frustrated so I banged my fist into the other hand and clenched it hard. "No," said the boy, "It's like this!" and he slapped himself repeatedly in the mouth and kept doing so until I mirrored him, only harder. A great smile came over his countenance. Finally, I had understood.

Often, following one of these symbolic mirrorings, the child will even put his feelings into words. "No, I'm not feeling sad. I'm feeling dirty. Make me an ugly face!" My histrionic ability leaves much to be desired. I'm not much of an actor. But somehow my deficiencies in this regard didn't seem to matter much, perhaps because the child always knew I was really trying to understand how he was feeling and, moreover, was accepting those feelings as being justified and natural. It was enough that for once he could experience those feelings without penalty or self-derogation. Again he learns that he is not alone, and again he feels the great relief that comes when unplesant feelings are shared with someone he can trust, a relief that results in more fluency.

Another procedure that I have used repeatedly involves projective drawings of the feelings evoked by stuttering. Both of us have a session in which we each draw pictures representing anger, fear, helplessness and so forth. Always the child draws something that he calls the "I am mad" or "I'm scared" face and one that shows a face scribbled all over, the "ugly" face for shame. But there are others too: one with a sad expression and tears, another with no mouth at all. One that I remember vividly was just a circle with two huge eyes in it. The child called it his "They're always looking at me" face, and it seemed to represent shame or embarrassment. One picture showed a baby sucking a bottle and the child used it to represent feeling little or helpless.

Sometimes a child will just scribble at random all over the card and will hold it up after a moment of stuttering to show that he doesn't really know how he feels except that he's all mixed up. After we have decided on the cards we want to use, I make a copy of them. Then when the child stutters, we both select the card that we think represents most closely his feelings at that moment and hold it up at the same time to see if we pick the same one. This procedure always stimulates verbalization of the feelings by the child if there are discrepancies. He feels impelled to explain why he chose that card and in the process often reveals many of the rejections and penalties he has received at home or at school. For example, after a long laryngeal blocking in which he struggled vainly to produce voice on a vowel word, one boy held up the card showing a face without a mouth and then let out one of the best primal screams I've ever heard. Then he said, "Maybe I ought to always yell like that when I get stuck. Like my Dad does at me!" These projective drawings of feelings related to stuttering moments are excellent pump primers.

Any clinician can devise other methods for helping young stutterers express in one way or another the feelings that trouble them. The important point, if any, in this little article is that clinicians should recognize the need for such venting in a permissive, caring situation and do something about it.

chapter four

Talking with Children Who Stutter

Dean E. Williams, Ph.D.

There is general agreement among most speech-language clinicians that some form of counseling is appropriate for adolescents and adults who stutter. There is not similar agreement, however, of its appropriateness for children of elementary school age. Often, there is disagreement about what counseling involves and how it can be "adapted" to children. Stated simply, counseling involves talking **with** another person. Of course a clinician **talks with** a child so the confusion must arise over the purpose of talking with them.

The purpose of talking with children who stutter is to discuss with them frankly and openly their beliefs about what they believe is wrong, what they believe helps them talk better, and what their feelings are about talking. Once this is determined, they need information about what talking involves and what they can do constructively in order to talk the way they want to talk. The talking that is done is structured around an active process of directing observations as the children are experiencing the ways they are talking and then of helping the children evaluate and re-evaluate their interpretations of those observations. The goal is to assist the children explore the reality of what they are doing and to introduce and demonstrate the alternatives they have for change. Said in another way, counseling is directed toward assisting children learn the elements of problem solving with regard to stuttering. To do this most effectively, clinicians cannot be indirect, cannot be coy and skirt around issues or topics, cannot assume the stereotype "teacher" role of **telling** the children what to learn, cannot talk "down" to them or on the other hand, adopt a "professional" language that is vague at best and scary at worst. Instead, a clinician should enter each child's language experience world and function from there. Most children will talk common sense with the clinician if the clinician will talk common sense with them.

Beliefs

Children who stutter generally receive much information about stuttering and many instructions of "what to do" or "what not to do" that are confusing and misleading. Before the clinician begins to explain the therapy program to a child, it is desirable to find out as much as possible about the child's beliefs about what his stuttering is. If this is not done, the child is likely to interpret the clinician's statements and therapy activities from a perspective of distorted and perhaps erroneous beliefs of what is wrong with his speech and what he perceives he has to do to improve. Hence, as clinical activities are presented and the child filters their purposes (as explained) through his own belief system, he is apt **to learn** things that are different from what the clinician intended **to teach.** Even though positive changes in speech are attained in the therapy room, the child's ability to transfer and to maintain them in all speaking situations becomes precarious when such changes are built on a foundation of the shifting sands of confused beliefs.

Talking with the children about what they **believe** is wrong and what they do that they believe helps them talk better can assist the clinician in providing meaningful information about the problem. Also, it assists in explaining the purposes of the proposed therapy program that are meaningful to a child — because they take into account the child's own view of the problem. Children differ in their beliefs as to what is wrong and what is helpful. Clinicians should be aware of this. Such awareness prevents them from falling into a ritualized "sameness" as they begin therapy with different children.

Most children's beliefs about why they have trouble talking (what's wrong) are often fragmentary and vague. Others just shake their heads and say that they don't know. Still others are quite imaginative and specific. Explanations from "words get stopped in my mouth" to "words get hooked in my throat on little fish hooks," deserve thoughtful consideration by a clinician as to their implications for what the children are trying to do as they talk to conquer the problem as they perceive it. Regardless of the reasons given by a child, they deserve and require respectful discussion with the child; not from a perspective of implying that the idea is silly or that it is wrong or that it is unimportant, but from the standpoint of listening, of questioning, of thinking out loud with the child what it means — of sharing with the child his dilemma. **No conclusions need be drawn at the time.** If the child seems to be confused or frightened by his uncertainties the clinician can reflect these or similar feelings by stating something like, "It's confusing isn't it?" Or, "It's kind of scary to not have any idea what's wrong isn't it? You're trying to talk and all of a sudden things just go whambo!" The clinician can terminate the discussion by stating something like, "Look, we'll come back and discuss this some more when we start talking about what you can do to help yourself improve the ways you talk."

The next area of beliefs to be discussed is **what the children have been doing to help themselves talk better.** If they have beliefs about what is wrong, the things they do to help ordinarily grow out of those beliefs of what is wrong. For example, the child who stated that "the words got hooked in his throat on little fish hooks," **pushed hard** in order to "slip the words off of the hooks" so he could "get them out." Clinicians should realize that children's beliefs create strong motivations for the ways they behave. If changes are attempted in the ways a person behaves without taking into consideration the motivations which prompt the behavior — even if changes are accomplished — they are apt to be unstable at best unless there are corresponding changes in the motivation for the behavior. This requires, often, an examination of the beliefs that are the guiding force for the motivation.

There are children who have no explainable reasons for what

they believe is wrong but few have no idea of what they can do to "help." Many of these ideas come from what they have been told by others. For example, two of the most common instructions they receive are "relax" and "slow down." The following conversations with children will illustrate the perplexing incongruity the children face between what they try to do to help, what they do, and their explanations for it.

First child in a conversation with the clinician.
Clinician: "So, you're talking along and all of a sudden you stutter. Why do you suppose it happens right there?"
Child: "Oh, I stutter when I talk too fast."
Clinician: "You do? How did you find that out?"
Child: "Well, when I stutter, they tell me to slow down."
Clinician: "Mmm-hmm, do they ever tell you to slow down when you don't stutter?"
Child: "No."
Clinician: "Why do you suppose they don't?"
Child: "I guess it's because I must be talking slower."
Clinician: "Oh, I see. Well, what do you do to help yourself when you talk?"
Child: "I try to slow down so I won't stutter."
Clinician: "Does that help?"
Child: "Some of the time."
Clinician; "Some of the time?"
Child: "Yeah. You see, I don't stutter all the time."

Second child in a conversation with the clinician:
Clinician: "You say you stutter some. What do you do to help at those times?"
Child: "I try to relax."
Clinician: "Oh, why do you do that — are you real tense?"
Child: "I don't know — they tell me to relax so I won't stutter."
Clinician: "Does it help?"
Child: "Yeah."
Clinician: "All of the time?"
Child: "Yeah, except when I stutter."
Clinician: "Mm-hmm. What do you do then?"

Child: "I just stutter."

Clinician: "And then what do you do?"

Child: "I just don't talk for a while."

Clinician: "You don't talk for a while, I see. Don't you feel like talking, or what?"

Child: "I feel kinda bad. I don't want to talk until I feel better."

Again, as with the earlier discussion, **there is no need for the clinician to confront and resolve the child's beliefs at the time.** The clinician, again, can reflect the child's feelings and possible confusion.

The example of the second child illustrates also how these ways of talking with a child open the door to discussing the child's feelings about stuttering and about himself. For younger children, the feelings are predominately ones of feeling "bad" or "sad." The overriding emotion is one of frustration. Strong embarrassment surfaces with many as they get older. The things they do to help are inconsistently helpful (according to their perceptions) or lead to more difficulty. An example of the latter is the child who said he helped by just pushing the word out. When asked what he did when that didn't help, he replied, "I push harder." They become frustrated because they are doing the only things they know to help themselves — and they are not too helpful. This leads to doubts about their ability to cope. They are experiencing conflicts about what to do. Things are not working the way they intended. They are developing feelings of helplessness. This is scary to them.

What's Going On?

When a clinician begins to share the particular view that the children have about what is wrong and what they can do to help themselves talk better, it should become obvious that the children need constructive information about what's going on. Stuttering appears to them to be very mysterious. They are confused by it. They are likely to feel that they are "defective" or that something is horribly "wrong with them." They can begin to feel that they are "dumb" or "incompetent" because they cannot overcome this "thing" by gritting their teeth and trying harder. After all, most adults seem to know how they can stop doing it. The children are told, for example, that if they would only "slow down" or "relax" or "think of what they are going to say" they wouldn't do it. It sounds so easy. Yet when they try it, they fail. There appears to be little, if any, relationship between what they do to help and the result of what they do. The trouble must be with **them.**

The clinician has a responsibility to each child to help him learn "what is going on" — what accounts for this disparity between what the child is trying to accomplish and the result. Or, said in a more constructive way, the clinician should help the child learn the relationship between what the child is doing to help and what he is doing to interfere with his speaking. Moreover, it should be done in ways that the child can understand. The word "understand" is used not to refer to a relatively abstract intellectual understanding, but to one based on the child's own world of experiences. He must be able to relate this "understanding" to his every day activities.

Too often, clinicians begin talking and philosophizing about stuttering by attempting to define it. This results in an explanation that includes the statement, "There are many different reasons given for stuttering. No one knows, for sure what causes it, but we'll do what we can to help you." This type of explanation easily can convey to the child that the clinician is as confused as he is, but something will be "tried." The compulsion that we have in our profession to discover "the cause" spills over into our clinical procedures. The child is not interested in the confusion among our stuttering theoreticians. He wants to know "what is going on" when he begins to talk and what he can do about it. This is reasonable. Instead of attempting to define stuttering, we need to **explain** to the child "what's going on" in a way 1) that reassures him that something terrible is not wrong with **him** and 2) conveys a positive direction involving constructive learning experiences.

My own personal preference is to explain it in terms of learning. The child is in the midst of the experiences of learning. He is learning at school, he is learning to get along with friends, he is learning, learning, learning. He knows what it means. Moreover, there is little doubt but that learning is **normal.** At the same time, it can be explained in ways that do not violate most responsible theories about the development of the stuttering problem. An example of the essentials of such an explanation follows:

Stuttering is a confusing thing to most boys and girls. It's tough to know what one can do about it. It seems at times it's almost like a "burp." You can feel it coming and, whoops, you burp! About the only thing you can do is press your lips tightly together so it won't sound too loud — or put your hand over your mouth so people won't notice it too much. Although stuttering may seem to be something like that, it really isn't. Stuttering is something you began to do when you were learning to talk. We all have to learn to talk — just like we have to learn to read or do arithmetic. When we learn, we make mistakes. That is a normal part of learning anything. It's true with learning to talk. (Examples are demonstrated of different types of disfluencies which make up the mistakes of talking.) It's no different from learning arithmetic. Some children make more mistakes than others when they learn arithmetic. Some make fewer. The same is true with reading — or with talking. But regardless, as we practice and learn, we get so we can do arithmetic, or read, or talk OK.

You probably made more mistakes when you were learning to talk than some of the other children did. You didn't want to make so many so you began to fight them. The harder you fought the more mistakes you made. It's kind of like learning to catch a ball. (Or any other similar type of behavior.) If you try hard to "not drop the ball" — or tense up and "pounce" at it so you won't goof, you drop it more often. This is the way it is when you do what we call "stuttering." You fight to say it right. When you fight, you tense, you may pounce (quick increase in velocity of movement). Or you may generally "hold back." When you do this you tense, maybe hold your breath and get set to "fight any mistakes you may make." This is a very normal reaction — a normal way to fight mistakes. You're OK. There is nothing inside you — in your mouth or throat or stomach that stops a word.

41

You learn to fight your speech. You can learn to talk smoothly.

The above explanation is **not presented in a monologue.** One includes the child in the discussion by asking if he understands, by asking for other examples, etc. Finally the clinician models different types of disfluencies, then asks the child to do them. Then the clinician models fighting them in different ways and asks the child to do the same. **This aspect may take several therapy sessions.** The child must experience them, explore them, puzzle over them as the clinician and child discover what he's doing. This then leads into comparing them with what he does during any "real" instances of stuttering. He needs to explore all the facets of the similarities and differences between the "fighting" he does in specified ways and the occurrence of a "real" stutter. The clinician needs to talk with him and examine them too. It's a period of learning, of discovery, of realization that **he is doing these things.** This is the foundation upon which the task of establishing congruence between intent and resulting behavior is learned.

The next necessary learning experience is to discover that as he changes the ways he "fights," he changes the result — or, the characteristics of the stutter. He should tense up more, then less. He should speed up velocity of movement, then decrease it, etc. He should talk and not fight so hard when he "stutters." The clinician should be involved by modeling the changes then asking the child to do the same thing. This establishes the foundation for **change.** It involves learning that the reality of changes is dependent on what the child **does.** This opens the door for improved self esteem, for the development of taking responsibility. The child can learn that **he** has something to do with what he does — and that what he does determines what "happens" when he talks.

The purposes of the activities described above should not be confused with those of "desensitizing to stuttering," or with those of "accepting one's stuttering." These are not designed to show the child that he should talk that way out in social situations. They are not therapy techniques aimed at the immediate production of fluency. **They are structured experiences designed in order to guide the observations the child is**

making. As he makes them, his perceptions and evaluations can be discussed with him. Different interpretations can be suggested by the clinician and then immediately tested. They can be **a most effective method of counseling with children regardless of the therapy procedures employed by the clinician to improve fluency.** It requires the child to discuss and evaluate his experiences in the reality of the present instead of from the unreality of his remembrances of the past.

The experiences and discussion described above will ordinarily bring to the surface the child's sensations of emotion. These can be shared and discussed openly. The clinician can lead such discussions in the direction of helping the child learn that attending and changing one's behavior is dependent on what the child **does** and is not dependent on reducing or eliminating one's emotions. He can learn that he can change the way he does things in the presence of emotion. This is one of the most effective ways for a child to cease depending on his "feelings" to tell him how he will talk. By so doing, the ways he "feels" becomes less important and what he does becomes more important during the process of talking. Hence, his **awareness** of "feelings" diminishes.

What Do We Do to Talk?

The question of "What do we need to do to talk?" naturally follows from — or blends into — the above discussion. For the clinician a more meaningful question is, "What does the child have to do to learn correspondence between what he intends to do and what he does?" Too often clinicians attempt to answer the question by imposing on the child a special speech pattern (either of fluency or of stuttering) in order, hopefully, to heal his wounded speech. This approach, it seems, reflects the clinician's limited perspective as much, or more, than it does the child's abilities or inabilities. Such an approach takes advantage, apparently without recognizing it, of the child's beautiful ability to cope and to adapt to a wide variety of ways of talking. Clinicians differ in what they preach and teach. Some extol movement, others air flow or relaxation, or slow movement, or smooth stuttering, or smooth transitions, etc., all with varying degrees of success. The wonderment of it all is that the poor child is able to cope with any or all of these cross-stitched sutures and still talk.

In order for the child to learn to be responsible for the ways he talks, it is important for him to problem-solve about what he does that helps him talk and what he does that doesn't help — in fact, what interferes with talking the way he intends. From his exploration of the behavior used to fight mistakes, he is aware that such things as tensing too much, holding his breath, etc., make talking difficult or impossible. It's time to learn what we do when we talk. This involves providing information about what the process of talking involves. "Providing information" does not include teaching him on an intellectual level the technicalities of speech production. It involves **explaining, demonstrating, experiencing** on a doing level the process of blending air, sound, movement, timing, tensing into the production of what we call words, phrases and sentences. Here the clinician can move each child's beliefs of what he thought was wrong and what he did to help (discussed earlier) into the reality testing arena for accuracy testing of his beliefs. Permit the child to test and discover for himself. Don't just **tell** him and expect him to "know it." If you do so, the child may know it intellectually but he won't know it in an operational-**doing** way. He needs to learn by experiencing that what we call a word is created primarily by a movement sequence of tongue, jaw and lips imposed on air or sound. Words don't come out of the throat or stomach. He needs to learn by experiencing the way we begin to talk — the initiation of movement with sound or air, the proper amount of tensing necessary, etc. This explanation cannot be done effectively at the level of words. The clinician leaves the level of words and relies on experiencing and doing — punctuated by words only to direct the observations that are to be more meaningfully experienced.

By experiencing the things necessary to do to talk the way he intends, it becomes meaningful to contrast these to different things he can do to interfere with the desired process. He can learn the relationship between tensing and increased velocity of movement, between restricting air and the production of sound, etc. In summary, he learns what we do to facilitate talking and what we do to interfere with it. Furthermore, he learns that stuttering is not something that erupts out of his mouth but, instead, consists of things he does to interfere with talking all along the vocal pathway. In addition, he learns that he **can** change what he is doing **as** he is talking so that it more nearly conforms to what he intends to do. By the continuous attending to the reality of what he is doing and knowing by experience what will help and what will hinder, he has the **time** to change in the ways he desires. This results in his learning that he has a choice. He is free to act in accordance with his choice. This is the goal of obtaining congruence between what a person intends and the way he behaves.

The intent of the approach to counseling through experience is to ensure in so far as is possible that the child can participate in a program to improve his fluency in a positive, matter-of-fact way. The counseling becomes an integral part of how the clinician helps the child to improve his speech. The child should possess the basic orientation that talking smoothly involves an active doing process to be learned — with the acceptance of the mistakes that accompany any learning.

chapter five

Talking with the Parents of Young Stutterers

C. Woodruff Starkweather, Ph.D.

Introduction

The parents of a child who stutters are naturally affected by the problem. They have understandable emotional reactions which may alter the child's environment and make the problem worse. Their attitudes help determine the family's communicative style. For these reasons, and because most parents want help in dealing with the problem, parent-counseling is important. Parent-counseling usually supplements direct therapy for the child, but often, particularly with preschool children, clinicians counsel parents without treating the child directly in an effort to modify the child's environment.

It is useful to approach parent-counseling with the attitude that change in the behavior and attitudes of adults is possible but often difficult. Clinicians who are aware of the difficulty have realistic expectations but can still convey a sense of optimism. Behavior and attitudes change through experience. Counseling leads parents to the kind of experiences that will help them change. These changes have two purposes: 1) to alter the child's environment so that his speech will improve more easily, and 2) to help the parents understand their child better.

Whatever changes occur in parents, they are changes begun and continued by the parents themselves. The clinician can suggest changes in the atmosphere of the home, in the parents' attitudes, or in their behavior, but only the parents themselves can bring about these changes. Parents influence their children in several ways. First, as models, parents demonstrate ways of talking and attitudes toward speech. Children are powerfully influenced by modeling and usually acquire the attitudes and behaviors of their parents. Second, parents establish rules which regulate home life — the background against which most of the child's talking occurs. Third, parents can be effective in directly modifying a child's speech.

The Clinician's Attitudes and Behaviors

There are certain clinician attitudes and behaviors that can help parent-counseling. One of the most delicate things clinicians do is convey judgments to the parents about their behavior. Most parents accept these judgments willingly, but it is easier for them when clinicians show that they have taken care in making judgments, if they are sensitive to the parents' and the child's feelings, and if they talk to the parents without being critical.

Much of parent-counseling consists of discussing the parents' and child's feelings about speech and stuttering. A good counselor can discuss emotional subjects openly but seriously, with the attitude that emotions are a serious and important part of life, but not so serious or delicate that they are "too hot to handle." Many people believe that emotions are built into a person's character and cannot be changed. Emotions can be hard to control, but they can change with increased understanding and awareness. Clinicians who believe this will find it easier to counsel parents.

The parents of young stutterers are often puzzled by some of the disorder's characteristics, and some of the clinician's time is spent providing explanations. This can be difficult because we know very little about the origins of stuttering. Effective counselors give explanations that satisfy the parents' needs without speculating or theorizing. For example, one of the things that puzzles parents is the way a child can talk fluently with one listener and then stutter very badly when talking to another. The parents may even believe that the child's "difficult" listeners are upsetting him in some way, or they may feel guilty or embarrassed that a particular listener always sees him stuttering so badly. Clinicians can explain that many aspects of speech change considerably from one listener to the next: vocal quality, vocabulary, syntax, pragmatics, rate, and rhythm. By pointing these changes out to parents, the clinician can help them understand that there are many possible reasons why a child's stuttering may fluctuate.

The Parents' Role in the Development of the Child's Self-Esteem

The child's sense of personal worth is an important part of his recovery to normal fluency, and there is much that parents can do to help the child increase it. One of the most powerful sources of influence is the parents' attitude toward their child. If they accept him as a person, he will consider himself worthwhile. If they don't give him enough time or attention, or fail to appreciate his best qualities, his sense of personal worth will be diminished.

From the beginning, the clinician evaluates the parents' acceptance of the child. There are no tests for this, but by talking to the parents about their child, the clinician can easily learn about their attitude towards him. The clincian's understanding, at first superficial, should develop quickly, and in time, the clinician should have a well-developed sense of how much the parents accept and appreciate their child.

This acceptance and appreciation can be increased. A good way to begin is to help the parents discuss and examine their feelings about the child. This step must be taken with care since social rules about what parents SHOULD feel about their children are consistent and universal — all parents should love their children completely and without reservation. But of course no one's feelings are so totally positive. A discussion of the child's qualities, good and bad, with the clinician encouraging the parents to examine and trust their feelings about the child is a starting point. Gradually, the parents may realize themselves, that their opinion of the child may be in certain respects a little low. With continued discussion their awareness, understanding, and acceptance of these feelings will develop. This leads to a second stage in which the goal of counseling changes. In this second stage, the goal is for the parents to learn to accept the child in spite of what they believe are his faults or shortcomings. This goal can be reached by continued discussion of the child's qualities, during which the clinician encourages (reinforces) statements and insights reflecting an appreciation of the child and calls to the parents' attention the appreciation of teachers, playmates, adult friends, and relatives.

It is always difficult to know for sure whether the changes that occur as a result of these sessions genuinely reflect the parents' attitude. With modeling of an attitude of appreciation, and with reinforcement for statements reflecting such an attitude, the parents will soon make the right kind of statements, but these statements may reflect only a very superficial change. Their sincerity will have to be judged from the parents' non-verbal communication, which is not always so easy.

The Role of Parents as Models

Parents play an important role as models in the development of a child's fluency. A few specific behaviors may be modeled directly, but indirect influences seem to be more powerful. From observing his parents, a child acquires attitudes toward speaking which in turn determine the way he talks.

One such attitude is the child's sense of time pressure. There is a certain amount of time pressure whenever we talk. We don't want listeners to lose interest. But time pressure can be too urgent, and this urgency may make a child disfluent. Parents can learn how to model behaviors and attitudes that will reduce the child's sense of time pressure, for example, by talking more slowly. If the parents talk very quickly, the child will learn to expect that information should be exchanged at a fast rate. Unevenness in the parents' speech rhythm also signals urgent time pressure to the child. Some variation in rate at clause and sentence boundaries is natural, but speech that slows way down after a clause or sentence to allow for thinking and then rushes madly forward signals to the child that ideas, once conceived, must be forced out as quickly as possible. During this hurried speech, disfluencies are likely to occur, take up more time, and increase the child's urgency, leading to struggle and avoidance.

Another modeling influence on the child's sense of time pressure is the parents' turn-taking style. The pace of a conversation, not the same as speech rate, is reflected in the amount of time that elapses between one speaker's turn and the next. Brisk turn-taking increases the child's sense of urgency about speech production, which may produce disfluencies which in turn he may struggle to avoid. Actual interruptions do this and more, informing the child that his thoughts are not appreciated.

The other side to this coin is that the child also learns to interrupt. It is hard for him to participate when the pace is fast and he has to interrupt or shout down someone else to get the floor. This competitive, verbal, fast-paced conversational style seems to be common in homes where the parents are well-educated and ambitious or where there are many older siblings. The young stutterer tries to enter the conversational fray. He has to try because in these homes it is clear that poeple are valued for what they can say. To get the floor successfully, the interruption must be well timed to occur during a lull in the conversation. And then, having successfully grabbed the floor, the young stutterer must immediately make a meaningful contribution. Of course he fails often. So, it is not just bad to interrupt the young stutterer, it is bad to require him to interrupt. Parents who interrupt and encourage verbal competition teach their children that they must interrupt and compete verbally in order to be appreciated.

Parents may also model a number of negative attitudes towards disfluency, their own or the disfluency of others. Fear, revulsion, impatience, or the idea that disfluencies are "errors" in speaking are a number of negative attitudes parents can have. Children quite naturally adopt these attitudes from seeing the parents react to disfluencies. This kind of modeling is probably most common in parents who stutter, but nonstuttering parents do this as well.

In a few cases, clinicians may find that parents are modeling avoidance behavior in response to problems other than stuttering or that their general approach to a problem is panicky and emotional. When this is the case and it appears that the child may be adopting this style and applying it to his speech in a way that increases struggle and avoidance, the clinician may want to counsel the parents about different ways to solve problems in general. In some more extreme cases of this sort, psychological referral may be required.

The Assessment of Parents' Fluency

When the parent of a young stutterer has speech that is too rapid, unusually disfluent, or shows signs of struggle or tension, clinicians may want to make an assessment of the parents' fluency.

Three observations can be made. First, the rate of the parents' speech can be assessed. Six syllables per second is rapid but normal. More than six syllables per second is fast. Second, the frequency of hesitations, interjections, stops/restarts, revisions, repetitions, and other disfluencies may be counted, and the time they take up may be measured. The number of disfluencies should seem appropriate for the topic and social setting. More important than the number of disfluencies is the parents' reactions to them, if any, and the attitude these reactions suggest. Finally, a rough assessment of tension or struggle to talk, or to talk fast, in the parents' speech should be noted. There are no formal assessment techniques, but it is not difficult to recognize in a speaker a sense of urgency to communicate.

Changing Parents' Fluency

There will be times when the clinician will want to try to change the parents' speech because of the modeling effects it is having on the child. If it looks as though it will be hard to modify parent's fluency, or if it has been tried without much success, clinicians should consider turning the child's attention to other models. The clinician is surely one. Relatives or friends whose speech is less rapid, or whose reaction to disfluency is more casual are others. Children who are a little older may be able to modify their speech patterns when their attention is turned to the speech of popular public figures. It is not wise, though, to present models whose speech is free of nonfluencies such as disc jockeys, professional speakers, or newsmen, who are usually too fluent and articulate to be appropriate models for a young stutterer. Often, they have trained themselves not to say "uh" or to hesitate at all. Sports figures may hit just the right note, displaying confidence, plenty of normal nonfluency, and a normal rate of speech.

When it is the parents' reactions to or attitude toward disfluency that the clinician wants to change, counseling or desensitization procedures may be used. Adult perceptions of disfluency and adult attitudes toward speech and disfluency are excellent targets for behavior change. In many cases too the motor speech patterns themselves are susceptible to counseling or behavior modification.

Reactions of Parents to Stuttering Behaviors

One of the primary goals of parent-counseling is a change in the way parents react when the child stutters. Parents should not be made to feel guilty over the way they react. Nearly all of the reactions parents have to stuttering are a direct result of the love and concern they feel for the child. Nor is it at all clear that these reactions in any way CAUSE the problem. But in many cases, the parents' reactions make the problem worse, or prevent its improvement, in spite of their good intentions. Clinicians who are experienced at parent counseling know that they can bring about change in parental behavior best by explaining that even though they didn't cause the problem, they are in the most powerful position to change the child's environment. A change in the child's environment may not, by itself, solve the stuttering, but it can allow other forces, such as the child's own development, or any direct therapy that may be going on, to have their fullest effect.

The kind of reactions that parents have which may prevent a child's fluency from developing are: pretending the stuttering doesn't exist, pained facial expressions, becoming very still during stuttering, expressing pity, inadvertent reinforcement for stuttering by paying attention or giving in to requests, expressing guilt over stuttering, intended or inadvertant punishment for stuttering, finishing sentences or supplying words, interrupting the child. No doubt there are many others.

Counseling may begin by making the parents aware of their reactions. Many parents have become so accustomed to reacting in a certain way that they do not even realize they are doing it or that it has any significance.

Videotapes and audiotapes of the parent and child talking together are a great aid in helping the parents become more aware of their reactions to the child's stuttering. As they realize how they react, they will often need to explain and justify the reactions. The clinician can be very supportive at this point, accepting the parents' motives. Parents can discover for themselves what the consequences of a certain pattern of reaction has been on their child's stuttering. This self-discovery provides the ideal motivation for behavior change. Once they clearly want to change, they will try to change their behavior consciously, and they may succeed. But often, the old pattern of behavior is hard to break. The clinician can help by suggesting two ideas. One is to attend to the child as a whole. Listen not so much to the child's speech as to his thoughts. What does he want you to know? Or feel? Another is to have the parents learn to focus on positive aspects of the child. Whatever attention they can focus on the child's good qualities will be attention turned away from his stuttering.

Things about Their Speech that Parents Can Change

Slowing Down the Conversational Pace and Removing Interruptions. Many parents need to have the ill effects of the fast-paced conversation that is full of interruptions explained to them. They don't realize the extent of the demands it places on their child, and they may not realize how the time pressure, coupled with the requirement for verbal excellence, works against fluent speech by simultaneously disrupting the flow of speech and demanding that the flow be as rapid as possible.

The clinician, in addition to explaining to the parents how such an atmosphere may affect the child's fluency, wants to achieve two other goals — a change in the conversational style of the home and and a motivation for the parents to make that change a lasting one. Changing the pace is relatively easy. All the parents have to do is wait before answering. Ask them to count to three before responding to another speaker. Other family members should also do this. It's easy to do, and slows the conversation immediately to a leisurely pace. The second goal is harder — motivating the parents and other family members to continue. For some families, the value of reflective thought may be extolled. An idea that has been considered, modified, and reconsidered is usually worth more than one that is just blurted out. For the family that seems to be rushing all the time, the serenity of a calmer life may be appealing. It often seems that people who cram every moment full of activity do not enjoy any of their activities very much. The family that is highly competitive may respond to the idea that every individual has inherent value and can be appreciated for whatever he has to offer. Finally, the family that is simply disorganized or rude in their conversational style may find it a relief to organize their conversations around some rules of common courtesy. This means not interrupting a speaker, but it also means not abusing the privilege of holding the floor by going on and on. If each speaker is mindful of the other's interests and desires, no one will talk for too long and everyone will have a chance to contribute at a relaxed pace. Of course, conversational habits are difficult to break and a period of adjustment is to be expected. Also, if artificial devices such as hand-raising, or a "moderator" have been used in the beginning, they should eventually be faded out.

Counseling and good motivation will probably succeed in slowing the conversational pace and eliminating harmful patterns of turn-taking. If, however, the family has developed a conversational style that is fast-paced, disorganized and competitive, the child will feel that he is competing with others in a verbal arena for which he is poorly equipped, a gladiator who has dropped his sword. The first thing to do to eliminate the ill effects of competition is to make sure that the child can get some time alone with his mother, his father, and with any other important family member who lives in the household. The second thing is to require that the family, when gathered together and talking as a group, refrain from any kind of evaluation of the contributions of others. This is only common courtesy anyway, but despite this it may be difficult to hold the family to it for very long if they are accustomed to frankly evaluating each other's contributions. Nevertheless, even if it can be adhered to only temporarily, it helps in reducing the child's sense of competing against all odds.

Eliminating "Demand" Speech. Few parents realize how difficult it is for a child to talk when he is told to "say 'thank you'" or "Tell Aunt Corinne what you saw at the zoo," or "Now tell me the truth!" Speech makes public the child's private self, and forcing him to talk requires him to do something that should be natural and spontaneous. Later in life he will acquire the knack of talking on demand. The forcing involved in demand speech is what makes children so shy about it. For children, these nonspontaneous modes of talking are difficult. Not asking it of them will help fluency develop.

Parental Attitudes Toward Speech Time. Although it is sometimes difficult for adults to change their speech rate directly, it is often easier for them to modify their attitudes toward speech time, which indirectly changes their rate. Several approaches are possible. Clinicians can show parents, by example, the value of taking the time to say what they really want to in the best way. By providing an example of speech that is not too fast and is well thought out, the clinician allows the parents to change by choice rather than by being told. Show them examples of public figures who are attractive and pleasant-sounding, whose speech is relaxed, self-assured, courteous, and not too fast. Many parents can appreciate a more leisurely attitude toward talking.

Attitudes toward Disfluency. By modeling an appropriate attitude, and by pointing out the disfluencies that exist in the speech of normal speakers, clinicians can help parents learn that disfluencies are not to be feared or avoided. Filled pauses, such as "um" or "uh," revisions, false starts, parenthetical remarks, and repeated words and phrases are not "errors" of speech but ways of gaining thinking time so that more accurately expressive words can be found. The content is more important than the form. In some few cases, parents may have to learn that disfluencies are not disgusting, painful to observe, or annoying in the speech of others. Nor do they reflect stupidity, carelessness, or nervousness. Instead they are a natural part of the process of language formulation, not only tolerable, but often desirable.

Reinforcements and Punishments for Disfluencies.   A careful self-examination of the parents' reactions to the child's disfluencies may uncover some reactions which constitute either reinforcement or punishment for disfluency. Videotaped or audiotaped interactions between parents and child are useful in uncovering these reactions. It is usually sufficiently motivating for the parents to become aware of these reactions and their possible consequences. With this awareness, the parents will almost surely alter their reactions. The danger is that they may alter their reactions too much or in undesirable directions. Many parents who discover that looking away or rolling their eyes at disfluencies signals displeasure begin to freeze instead, or change the subject. These reactions are just as bad. Most helpful is to teach parents to listen to what their child has to say rather than to how he says it. This gives them something to do, something to react to, instead of simply telling them not to react in a certain way.

Willingness to Talk about Stuttering.   Finally, but probably most important, parents can break the conspiracy of silence and become willing to talk openly about stuttering, to answer the child's questions about it, to explore it with the child. Just how this is done depends on the child's age and level of understanding and on the extent of the child's own willingness to talk about it. With a younger child, it is simply a matter of answering his questions at the level he seeks understanding. For the older child who has stopped asking, clinicians will find it most helpful to sit down with parents and child and begin. Present the session as an opportunity to ask questions about stuttering. Encourage discussion. It won't be long before the topic is open again.

Conclusion

Much can be done through parent counseling to help the stuttering child. Attitudes and behaviors of the parents and of the rest of the family can be modified in ways that help the child develop normally fluent speech. Parent-counseling can help to remove barriers which hinder the child's treatment, barriers that may undo at home the clinician's work in the therapy room.

Clinicians who counsel successfully begin from the premise that parents feel acutely responsible for their children's behavior, and this includes stuttering. It often seems to be the case that this sense of responsibility, in its more extreme forms of anxiety, guilt, and frustration over stuttering may have contributed to the problem, but this is obviously not an idea that should be conveyed to the parents. In fact we don't know what causes stuttering. Nor should there be suggestions from the clinician that parents have made the problem worse or prevented the child from developing normal speech. These ideas will only increase the parents' guilt, frustration, and anxiety, and many parents will already have come to believe that the child's stuttering is their fault. It is helpful to tell parents that they offer the best hope for positive change. Their frequent presence and their concern make this evident. Suggestions can be made effectively without damaging their sense of authority. The decision to do something is left to them so that when they act, they will do so with a strong personal conviction.

chapter six

Stuttering vs. Fluency

William H. Perkins, Ph.D.

Punishing as stuttering can be, it nonetheless can have its own peculiar rewards. A function of counseling is to help stutterers confront the reality of how they feel about the price of stuttering, its payoffs, and its role in their self-concepts. Failure to cope effectively with these feelings can seriously impede permanent improvement of speech.

Payoffs

The price of stuttering is so visible as to make the struggles of speaking seem painful. On the face of it, what could anyone find rewarding about stuttering? Yet from its earliest occurrences, reinforcements are likely to begin accumulating. Typical ones derive from the success with which parental attention is obtained. Parents of children who stutter tend to become sensitized to the problem. When this happens, their attention is more likely to be commanded by stuttered than fluent speech.

That stuttering apparently can continue to command attention as the child matures to adulthood seems probable. In one instance in which a severe stutterer achieved fluency quickly, panic ensued with the discovery that conversational command would depend on the importance of what he had to say instead of on the automatic attention his struggles to speak had provided.

A variety of other benefits can be acquired by the time a person who stutters reaches adulthood. Some are so apparent that stuttering is turned on or off as the occasion demands: the lady whose husband thinks she's sexy when she stutters a bit, entertainers whose careers are built on stuttering, the young man whose girl friends think his stuttering is attractive. Less obvious was the aging lumberjack who stuttered on virtually every syllable, sometimes for over a minute. After obtaining fluency with a very slow rate, he resisted speeding up. The reason turned out to be that he had trouble thinking at the new rate, slow as it was, because it was so much faster than his stuttered rate with which he had become comfortable over the years.

The foregoing payoffs are not always readily apparent, but they do not lurk far below the surface. Extensive counseling is not needed to reveal them. Subtler, more pervasive, and probably more powerful payoffs develop in the self-concepts that can evolve. Stuttering was observed in more than fifty adult stutterers during some 4,000 hours of counseling and psychotherapy. Its central value for these people was that it seemed to protect them from a feeling of loss of impact. Who has not experienced this feeling in conversation which seem to flow over us, around us, and through us as if we did not exist? A shield that would protect us from this sense of worthlessness would have immeasurable value. Stuttering can provide such a shield.

One manifestation is that it makes possible an idealized identity in which the stutterer can be unlimited in the imagined powers he has. In effect, he says to himself that if he did not stutter, he would be a giant. As a young minister said of his speech, "It's like I'm constantly painting masterpieces. Of course I know they aren't real masterpieces, but they feel like it inside. The only way I can protect them is to spoil them with stuttering so people won't know for sure that they weren't masterprieces."

Curiously, this problem has an opposite side. When stripped of their protective shield, some have had relief from stuttering. An accountant who never blocked with his subordinates but always had difficulty with his supervisors suddenly reversed this pattern. A month earlier, a new supervisor had taken over and had insisted on things being done to his specifications. As the accountant reported, "I finally have given up. I know this guy isn't going to listen to me regardless of how good my reasons are. When I'm talking to him I feel like a useless blob, but for some reason I don't stutter with him anymore. Now though, when I have to tell the people working under me to do things his way, I get all tied up." It is possible to speculate that stuttering functioned to protect his self-concept. When it was deflated and while he had nothing left to protect, perhaps he had no need to stutter, or perhaps it was because communicative stress was reduced.

Stuttering can also shield against unsatisfactory personal relations. Here is how a writer described this problem. "I seem to be the only one who feels affection, but my anger isolates me even more from the people I want to like me, so I live in my warm private inner self where I can feel perfect and stay away from the cold barren outside world. The only way I can enter that world is when I'm in communication with someone who makes me feel that I'm everything in reality that I secretly am inside. I guess I try to be as perfect in real life as I am in my daydreams in the hope that people will be impressed and give me the approval I need, but of course I can't because I stutter."

Psychotherapy

From this discussion you may have concluded that psychotherapy is essential to the successful treatment of stuttering. Extensive experience suggests, though, that psychotherapy is more useful as an adjunctive means of preserving improvements achieved with speech therapy than as the primary mode of treatment. Were stuttering a symptomatic resolution of psychoneurotic conflict, then it should yield to psychotherapeutic resolution of the conflict. Rarely does this happen, although when it does, the people for whom psychotherapy has been effective are likely to think of themselves as "cured."

When ego-protective payoffs interfere with progress, they may require psychotherapy. More typically, however, the conflicts in need of resolution seem more a consequence than a cause of stuttering. These conflicts can be as intractable as if they were psychoneuroses from which stuttering sprang. To attack them, however, with psychotherapy as the primary treatment of choice is to engage in a form of therapy whose effectiveness cannot be adequately tested without a major investment of time, money, and effort. Accordingly, alternative counseling tactics have been developed.

Improving Self-Esteem

Based on the premise that success breeds success, an experiential form of counseling is used. Clients learn through doing that self-defeating assumptions and attitudes are unnecessary and, indeed, are false. These take two major forms: 1) helplessness to change how they speak and how people react to them, and 2) conviction that most of their problems would be solved if they did not stutter.

Helplessness to change can be dealt with by establishing normally fluent speech, or by gaining control of moments of stuttering that relieves them of helpless struggle. Both provide clear evidence that speech fluency is not mystical, but is behavior which can be altered and controlled.

Assignment of one's problems to stuttering is probably easier to resolve with normal fluency than with struggle-free stuttering. Although neither "cures" the stutterer, being able to sound like a normal speaker helps enable him to face the reality that his other problems still exist.

In fact, it was to achieve resolution of this second problem in an artist being seen for psychotherapy that a rate-control program for fluency was developed in the first place. This young man insisted that his woes, and there were many of all sorts, were entirely a consequence of his stuttering. This false conviction undermined psychotherapeutic progress, so fluency was established to demonstrate that freedom from stuttering did not dissolve his problems. Ironically, with his defenses exposed, the artist eventually protested that he would rather stutter than drone fluently. He quit therapy and went off on his own to solve the problems on which he had refused to work in psychotherapy. Within two years, he not only was fluent but no longer considered himself a stutterer. This is not a testimonial for an atypical success of misfired psychotherapy but rather for the power of behavioral confrontation to alter false assumptions.

At least for those stutterers who have chosen a therapy which establishes fluency, the biggest problem they will encounter is with its maintenance. To solve this problem will often require solution of the feelings of helplessness and of the ego-protective values of stuttering just discussed.

Following is a direct intervention approach that can be used along to facilitate personal adjustment or can be used in conjunction with traditional counseling and psychotherapy. Rather than attempting to improve attitude as a prelude to improving speech, achievement of fluency is used as a basis for improvement of attitude.

Cost-Effectiveness

Maintenance of improvement, certainly of fluency and probably of struggle-free stuttering as well, is viewed as a problem of cost-effectiveness. Cost is measured in effort expended to maintain progress. (Financial cost does not appear to have much effect on long term success of therapy.) Effectiveness is measured in the various subjective terms that contribute to strengthening or weakening the importance of fluency. Freedom from punishment of stuttering, enjoyment of being fluent, and need for fluency at work and home strengthen the effectiveness side of the ratio; payoffs of stuttering such as those discussed above weaken it.

Self-Management

In so far as possible, the request for an initial interview should come from the person seeking help, not from a spouse, friend, parent, or employer. Success of therapy depends on concentration and diligence. A person who begins treatment for reasons other than strong personal need virtually ensures eventual failure.

Throughout treatment, either self-management or dependency will be fostered by the manner in which each clinical step is offered. Steps presented as requirements to be met place the clinician in the role of drill sergeant responsible for marching the client through therapeutic paces. The same steps that meet the same performance criteria can foster client responsibility when presented as options to be elected. In this approach, the clinician's task is to clarify the requirements of the step, the reasons for it, and the alternatives to not taking it, which may include termination of therapy, at least temporarily. In this vein, therapy proceeds by "ifs": "If this is what you want, then this is what you will need to do." The decision to take the step or not to take it is left with the stutterer.

A goal of self-management is to exorcise magic and mysticism from both fluency and stuttering. But the cost exacted can seem high. Attention to speaking skills is generally necessary, and the more severe the stuttering, the greater the likelihood that attention to these skills will remain a longstanding requirement of improved fluency. Assumption of responsibility for the choice of stuttering or being fluent acknowledges that both are forms of behavior subject to volitional control. To establish and maintain fluency, or to extricate oneself from stuttering once fluency is disrupted, usually requires voluntary use of various fluency skills.

For those who value control of their lives, the merits of self-management are lucidly apparent. Whether one wishes to stutter or to speak fluently becomes a matter of rational choice between the benefits of fluency and the price of attention to fluency skills. Rather than stuttering being a "thing" visited unwanted on the stutterer, it becomes a form of behavior that can be permitted, prevented, or modified. With self-management, both fluency and stuttering are for the stutterer, of the stutterer, and by the stutterer.

Realistic Expectations of Therapy

Judging from published and unpublished reports of fluency shaping programs, the most predictable outcome is regression of varying amounts and durations. Some progress is typically retained, but the expectation of permanent fluency is an expectation rarely realized. Those clinicians may well be correct who warn their clients that fluency is permanently theirs if they will constantly use the skills that are taught. The reality is that precious few are willing or able to do so. Sadly, those severe stutterers who most need to use the skills to preserve any vestige of fluency are the ones most likely to tire of the effort and to relapse fastest and farthest.

The programs offer skills which will provide freedom of choice between stuttering and fluency are alternatives to programs that offer fluency as an outcome of therapy. The emphasis is not on stutter-free speech but instead on mastery of skills by which such speech is available. This is accomplished by explicit counseling of what to expect from therapy, and more importantly, by what the clinician values during treatment. Greeting fluency with enthusiasm and stuttering with disappointment, to say nothing of extolling the virtues of fluency, speak loudly to the expected outcome of therapy. By contrast, the clinician can demonstrate by her attitude that the objective of therapy is mastery of skills (such as control of rate, of breath flow, of rhythm) of which fluency will be a by-product. The importance of skills — as opposed to fluency — will also be revealed directly in the attention given to measurement and evaluation of each specific ability being learned.

Without effective tools for recovery, the cost of relapse following treatment is especially devastating, which is why therapy that lasts a weekend is dangerous. True, fluency is easily obtained within hours, if not minutes. But mastery of the skills to maintain it in daily life typically requires extensive concentration, practice, and refinement of performance. The risk of any program that provides fluency without the support skills to maintain it is that clients will, probably, have learned what to do to remain fluent without acquiring the facility to do it. This leads to the cost of perceptual distortion and guilt. If the clinician is blamed for the client's failure to be as fluent as expected, then his improvement, which may be considerable, can be diminished or even denied. Conversely, if the clinician is esteemed, clients will often blame themselves for the discrepancy between the fluency expected and the fluency achieved. Some will tend to resolve this by perceiving their fluency as being better than it is. Worse, they will assume responsibility for failure to be as fluent as they expected so, worse yet, their guilt will isolate them from seeking further help.

The benefits of counseling the stutterer about realistic expectations of therapy are more likely to be long term than short. Most who enter a fluency-shaping program are probably attracted by the enticement of stutter-free speech. Doubly attractive is the prospect of fluency after only a few days of treatment. The honeymoon with fluency, during which use of fluency skills seems a small price to pay, typically lasts a month or two. By then, the realization of the price to be paid has dawned. Those who will tire of the "marriage" to fluency will begin to sort out from those who are willing to pay the price.

Thus, stressing reality of treatment outcome offers the major benefit of reducing the fluency "divorce" rate.

Realistic Expectations: Relapse vs. Fluency

Maintenance programs generally continue transfer activities, but on a less intensive basis. Two approaches are typically used, but both emphasize the value of fluency. One is to provide supervised practice in the maintenance of fluency. Some evidence, thought it is not definitive, suggests that permanence correlates with the number of hours of treatment, so there is merit in this approach. Undoubtedly, automatization of fluency, or any skill, is improved with practice.

The other approach can be harmful. The lure of fluency can be as tempting for clinicians as clients. To seek fluency for one's own reasons is one thing, but to be exhorted to fluency explicitly or implicitly by someone else is quite another. Such exhortation comes in several forms: pressure to use fluency skills, discussions of the merits of fluency, inquiries into adequacy of motivation. The worst source of all is from clinicians. They have labored mightily to help clients improve, sometimes dramatically. They can easily invest themselves heavily in that improvement. Sensitive clients work diligently for their clinicians, and their guilt is proportional to their sensitivity when industrious monitoring wanes and fluency slips.

Clinicians, like parents, who work to free their charges of dependence are no less dedicated than those who, out of their concern, inadvertently foster dependence. Clients of clinicians for whom fluency is a self-evident blessing will likely feel that they should be working for fluency whether they wish to or not. The preferable alternative is to offer the opportunity to learn the tools that will provide freedom of choice.

A basic condition for freedom, which clinicians control, is that each step of therapy from beginning to end be taken as a free choice by the client. Every step taken as a mandate is a step into dependence on the clinician. Therapy becomes something done **to** the client instead of **for** the client. To foster self-management, the clinician's responsibility is to present each step as an option, with all of the information and support needed to proceed successfully. The final decision to take or not to take the step, and the rate at which it is taken, is made exclusively **by**

the client. Admittedly, this ideal is more difficult to achieve in group than individual therapy. Nonetheless, better that each step be taken as a choice of the group than of the clinician.

A more tangible procedure in preparation for relapse is to arrange to have clients enter all of the feared conditions under which they expect to have difficulty. Until they have demonstrated to themselves that they can use their fluency skills successfully in every situation in which they have anticipated stuttering, the clinician's responsibility is not complete. Freedom to choose between fluency and stuttering exists only for those clients who have proven to themselves that fluency skills will work successfully in any situation **in which they elect to use them.**

A final procedure, perhaps most important of all, is that clients gain facility in using their fluency skills to recover from stuttering. The prospect of relapse of some extent or another is too great to assume that ability to recover will not be needed. Recovery practice involves two major activities. First is an analysis of the stuttering to discover which of the fluency skills are managed inadequately when stuttering occurs. The reason, of course, is to objectify and demystify stuttering so that the behavior of it is as much available to voluntary control as is the behavior of fluency. Second is practice in recovering from stuttering. This requires **reversing** those skills that provide fluency, such as increasing rather than decreasing speaking rate, until stuttering occurs. An alternative procedure is to have clients analyse their videotapes of stuttering as a basis for simulating it.

These recovery activities should not begin until mastery of fluency skills provides assurance of normal fluency. It is confidence in the knowledge that fluency is readily available that makes voluntary relapse feasible. Relapse without such certainty is understandably frightening. What has been learned is fluency as an alternative to stuttering. There is fear that if stuttering recurs, fluency will be lost forever. Until the recovery step is taken, clients do not have first hand knowledge that they do indeed have freedom of choice. It is the exercise of this choice between stuttering and fluency that should be practiced in every aspect of transfer, maintenance, and daily life.

These preparations for relapse involve at least three costs. One is that the bright expectation of permanent fluency is tarnished with dull reality. To prepare for relapse instead of for fluency seems, on the face of it, to be a denial of the whole purpose of therapy. Another cost is the requirement that the behavior of stuttering be confronted squarely. Many stutterers feel that it is too painful to face, an attitude which contributes to their impression that when it occurs, they have lost control. Finally, the procedure of transferring mastery of fluency skills to all feared conditions requires facing these conditions. Included in this price is willingness to forego the various techniques, such as avoidance devices, for preventing stuttering. Reliance on these can be so great that to contemplate relinquishing them amounts to inviting the recurrence of stuttering.

Preparation for relapse reduces the cost of constant vigilance. Conviction based on demonstrated ability to stutter and return to fluency frees clients of the necessity of maintaining fluency continuously. Without such confidence, fear that uncontrollable stuttering will return lurks behind breaks in the flow of speech.

What is offered is not management of moments of stuttering. Unlike pullouts and preparatory-sets, which are intended as devices to remove the struggle from stuttering, relapse recovery procedures are used to reestablish a normal flow of fluent speech which is free, not only of stuttering, but of "stickiness" of impending stuttering.

With this approach, a full range of options is available. Those for whom continuous fluency is important can have it by paying whatever price in monitoring and use of fluency skills is required. This price will vary from person to person, and probably from time to time. Similarly, the same price is required of those for whom rapid automatization of fluency is important. The premise for this price is that each relapse provides a refresher course in precisely those disfluent behaviors that the client is attempting to replace.

But for those whose determination to be free of stuttering fluctuates (which, in our experience, is the vast majority) the option of fluency is not lost or jeopardized by occurrence of periods when the price is too high. With confidence born of repeated successful recoveries under even the most feared of conditions, stuttering and fluency can be deciduous, each being shed and regained according to the cost-effectiveness ratio of the season.

chapter seven

Principles of Therapy

Joseph G. Sheehan, Ph.D.

All of us go through life meeting role expectations, or trying to meet them, sometimes succeeding, sometimes failing. When we fail publicly, we are shamed. When we fail privately in meeting our own self-expectations, we experience guilt.

Shame

Shame is an obvious occurrence in the disorder of stuttering, for the stutterer is expected to speak, and to speak fluently within normal limits, and fails to do so. In the process, he may exhibit behavior that listeners find mystifying and repellant, for talking always seems simple to those who have forgotten how complex the skill was to acquire in the first place. To understand the disorder as clinicians, we need to experience these audience reactions, often by acquiring the role of the stutterer with whom we are working so that we can know a part of what he experiences as he tries to speak but blocks instead. In the process, we may also experience a reaction of having done something wrong, of failing to do justice to ourselves and to our listeners. Like the stutterer, we can experience guilt, the private anguish that stems from the feeling that we haven't done right, or haven't measured up.

Guilt

The part played by guilt in stuttering can hardly be over-estimated. It is likely that feelings of guilt lie heavily in the background of the onset of stuttering, help to maintain the behavior once started, and tremendously complicate the whole process of therapy and counseling the stutterer.

The impact of guilt on fluency may be observed even in normal speakers. When confessing something, or defending our own actions, or offering explanation under threat, none of us is likely to remain smoothly fluent. In the stutterer, guilt heightens fear, or multiplies with fear to undermine fluent word production. We reduce fear for the stutterer by decreasing his feeling that he is doing something wrong every time he stutters. This is what we mean by acceptance of the problem, of the stutterer role to a sufficient degree that the problem may be discussed, analyzed, and worked on in a healthy and open atmosphere.

We may distinguish among several kinds and possible sources of guilt reactions in the stutterer. Some of these are relived each time the stutter blocks on a word, and may contribute to the mixture of shame, relief and guilt many stutterers experience upon release of the word.

Sources of Shame and Guilt

1. Primary guilt refers to the constellation of feelings that preceded and led to the appearance of blocking speech in the first instance. For example, a child of two may have been negated and shamed so often that he is profoundly uncertain about trying speech at all. Speech reflects attitude toward oneself, among other things. If a young child has been made to feel that he is often wrong in everything, he easily comes to feel that he is wrong in his fumbling efforts to acquire the speaker role.

2. Secondary guilt stems from not fulfilling expectations to speak, once the stuttering behavior has emerged. The constant suggestions of neighbors and strangers to the stutterer to take a deep breath, to think what he has to say, to slow down, to try some trick — all these imply that stuttering is a simple problem with an easy solution if the stutterer will just follow the proffered advice. But usually, the stutterer has tried them all, failed with them all, and each reiteration of the suggestions merely adds to his frustration and despair. Morever, there is a role expectation of immediate improvement tied to these bits of advice. When the stutterer has to reject them, he feels guilty. When he tries them and they fail, he feels guilty. "When I Say No, I Feel Guilty," is the title of a popular book on assertion training. One of the book's suggestions for overcoming feelings of guilt and inadequacy is the technique of "Broken Record," a courteous but firm and persistent statement of what you really want. It is far more therapeutic to fulfill your own aspirations and expectations, rather than those of others.

3. Audience punishment guilt stems from the stutterer's realization that his struggling and grimacing speech is distressing and punishing to his listeners — or to his projection that his stuttering behavior is punishing to others. This is qualitatively different from merely feeling that you didn't measure up to fluency demands. Although there seem to be a few stutterers so neurotic as to derive sadistic satisfaction from punishing audiences, they are not typical. Moreover, even those individuals can feel guilt along with the dubious satisfaction of having punished their audience along with themselves.

Research has well established a positive relationship between threat or expectation of penalty, and frequency of stuttering. We tend to stutter most where it hurts most. Ironically, it is often the case that the audience isn't nearly as concerned or as punished as the stutter assumes or projects. Discussion of the stuttering problem with the clinician and observational assignments may greatly reduce the stutterer's guilt and concern about punishing the audience. Most stutterers in therapy come eventually to realize that the damage they imagine they have been doing to listeners is like the premature reports of Mark Twain's death — greatly exaggerated.

4. Therapy-induced guilt is the fourth discernible kind, and it has profound effects on the course of therapy, and the counselor's relationship to the stutterer. The implied or explicit contract with the stutterer calls for greater fluency, at least eventually. Every clinician wants to help the stutterer speak better — that's the reason the stutterer is there. But there is a great hazard in premature expectations. Many a promising stutterer, in terms of response to therapy, has bogged down over the knowledge that he is expected to improve soon. Where the pressures for fluent performance are scheduled ahead of the time the stutterer can get ready to deliver, a clinical failure and consequent guilt may ensue.

Readiness for change is a central element in all therapies. But not every person who comes, is sent, or is brought into therapy has a readiness to change. For example, many stutterers have well-stabilized patterns of retreat and subterfuge, and aren't about to give them up without hefty resistance. As clinicians or counselors, we need to sharpen our ability to estimate the factor of readiness, so that we don't push when the client is not ready to move. At least, we don't push beyond his limits and receptiveness, or he may become so frustrated and guilty that he drops out or regresses rather than progresses.

Some degree of therapy-induced guilt is built in to the whole venture of therapy. Nearly all therapies currently in use call for the stutterer to be an active participant to some degree. He has to do something besides just talk. Under these conditions, it is easy for the stutterer to feel guilty over not **doing** enough. If the clinician has unwittingly encouraged the common belief on the part of the stutterer that perfect, stutter-free speech must be the goal, the burden of guilt can never go away. Speech need not be letter-perfect, or fluency-perfect, in order to be acceptable. Even accomplished actors will flub at times. In fluency as in many other things, perfectionism is a self-defeating goal. Any persisting feeling on the part of the stutterer that he has failed on any dimension of therapy will tend to undermine the self-worth upon which fluency must be based.

5. Clinician-induced guilt. We have been discussing therapy-induced guilt, that is, feelings in the stutterer that develop from his awareness that he has not done enough, that he did not meet role-expectations he had set up for himself. The stutterer may have some underlying mistrust of the therapist and the procedures he offers — and the feeling is often mutual. In this atmosphere lurks ample opportunity for self-blame and for other-blame. We have called the self-blame kind therapy-induced guilt; it develops naturally and inadvertantly. But some clinicians, deliberately or otherwise, induce guilt and shame reactions more directly. As an excuse for a program or clinician failure, they choose to manipulate the stutterer's already strong guilt and shame readiness. After weeks or months of therapy with repeated relapse, they put an ironic twist on the idea of acceptance. Finally they say or imply to the stutterer, "After all, remember that you're a stutterer, and you might as well accept that fact."

Acceptance of the problem belongs at the start of therapy, not at the finish. It is the role that the stutterer must accept, not the old stuttering pattern. That is what the stutterer entered therapy to eliminate! If he should be asked to accept the old pattern, then he should have been asked not to undertake therapy. To promote "acceptance" at the end of the venture to excuse clinician failure or method failure is an outrage. We need not accept what we can change — and the stutterer can change. If the stutterer had wanted to "accept" not for the purpose of enabling change, but in order to remain as he was when he came in, then he would not have come. When a clinician heaps blame on the stutterer at the end of therapy, then the client's hopes have been abused.

6. Timing as a source of guilt. As in any counseling relationship, the mishandling of the factor of readiness for change can lead to guilt and a vague sense of failure. Timing is crucial, for it reflects the sensitivity and competence of the clinician. An expectation to perform at a certain level at one stage may be less appropriate at another. Perfectly good procedures may be inappropriate depending upon the readiness of the person. For example, some discussion of the problem is endemic to virtually all therapies, even if only to spell out the arrangements. Some stutterers are just not ready to tolerate even that much self-confrontation. Even the discussion of the problem with the counselor may be painful. Skill in counseling persons who stutter requires an ability to recognize discomfort signs, and to see that therapy-induced guilt does not lead to discouragement, low morale and premature termination.

Stuttering Coexists with Other Problems

Many other problems may coexist with the problem of stuttering, and the clinician needs to be equipped to help the stutterer with these problems, within reasonable limits. Becoming a person who stutters does not exempt anyone from becoming a person with many other problems. It should not be assumed that the guilt and inadequacy feelings often shown by those who stutter are entirely the result of the stuttering. As one example, a stutterer may seem depressed, and it would be easy for him — and the clinician — to assume that he is depressed **because** he stutters, or that he stutters because he is depressed. But the relationship of these factors cannot be assumed — they may be connected or not, or they may be connected but only minimally. As another example, a stutterer may be either hostile or pervasively anxious; but might he not be either of those things whether he stuttered or not? Such feelings might easily **not** be associated with his stuttering. Because in individual cases, hostility might be evidently connected with stuttering, does not mean that it must be psychodynamically related in each and every case. The relationship of stuttering to coexisting problems is largely unexplored territory, and this question is left unanswered by those studies merely comparing stutterers with control groups. In individual diagnosis the relationship of other problems to the stuttering must often await their emergence during the course of therapy. Problems that will effect the later course of therapy often fail to surface during the initial interview.

As clinicians we sometimes need to remind ourselves that we are treating a person, not just a case of excess disfluency. In some clinics the stuttering group is called the "fluency group," apparently on the premise that fluency is the sole problem and the only goal worth mentioning. Many clinicians could facilitate the path toward fluent utterance more effectively by helping the person feel better about himself in all his roles in life, not just his speaking role.

A stutterer may feel ugly or lonely or unwanted or excluded from the mainstream of meaningful interaction with other human beings, and these feelings would all tend to contribute to the haltingness of his speech. But we cannot assume that he has these feelings only because he stutters. He might have them anyway. Nor can we assume that even a successful behavioral treatment of the stuttering would automatically remove all these feelings of self-doubt and inadequacy. By thinking only in terms of stuttering behavior, the clinician may overlook an opportunity to help the stutterer with other significant problems.

The "Giant in Chains" Complex

The stutterer himself often thinks that if only he did not stutter, he would have no other problems, and there would be no end to his accomplishments. We have called this the "giant in chains" complex — the feeling that if only we did not have that problem, nothing else would be wrong. Awareness as clinicians of the overattribution of all problems to the stuttering may help us avoid the same illusion so frequently held by stutterers, or by persons with any kind of handicap.

Nearly every stutterer has heard of the legend of Demosthenes, the Greek who overcame a speech impediment and became a great orator. It becomes almost a role-expectation. Yet we know that stutterers typically do not become great orators, even when they recover, with or without therapy. This is the "Demosthenes Complex."

The "giant in chains" idea is much broader. It refers to the overattribution on the part of the stutterer of all significant problems to the stuttering, to the handicap. If only he did not stutter, then there could be no limit to his accomplishments. Here is a defensive function that can cause reactions of disappointment to the stutterer as he begins to improve. Unless we are aware of it, we may not realize that improvement brings many problems with it, and that there is a process of adjustment to fluency.

Respecting Feelings

In stuttering we deal with both feelings and behavior, with both classically conditioned and instrumentally conditioned patterns of response. As clinicians we need to be aware of the distinction between these two classes of response, for they require some different handling in therapy. On the feeling level there must be no right or wrong. If a stutterer feels fear or shame or guilt, then help him to explore those feelings, for they may relate crucially to his stuttering and to his attitude toward himself and others, and toward speaking in the world. On the feeling level, the "shoulds" and "should nots" must not apply. Otherwise the person who stutters will tailor his disclosure of feelings and attitudes toward what he imagines the clinician wants to hear. Feelings have a validity of their own, and should be respected.

Altering Behavior

On the doing level it may be different. Stuttering behavior is full of instrumental or operant responses: for example, grimaces, head jerks, sudden forcings or increases in muscle tension, and the like. These are the "tricks" that are so evident to the audience and so handicapping to the stutterer. As operant responses, they are determined by their consequences. If the consequence of using a head jerk is the sudden release of the word the stutterer has been trying to say, then this operant response will increase in frequency. Put differently, we increase the behaviors that seem to pay off. However, for the stutterer it is only a temporary and unreliable payoff. Next time it may not work, either due to a decrease in the novelty of response-produced stimuli, or because the interpersonal situation may be less favorable. On the level of behavior while speaking, there are some "rights" and "wrongs" for the stutterer. The clinician may be accepting and forgiving of the stutterer's feelings and fears, but he cannot be equally neutral about the stutterer's behavior while trying to speak. Operant responses do have consequences, and those consequences determine the pattern of future behavior of the same kind.

For example, the stutterer may tap his foot to get a word out, and the behavior may appear to be successful, for lo and behold, the word does emerge. The stutterer may offer himself premature congratulations, for he has just become more dependent on an unreliable friend. Some stutterers even brag about fooling listeners or using tricks successfully, although for most, a profound guilt is more common. It is both a right and a duty for the clinician to point out the relationship of such intermittently successful operant responses to the visibility of the handicap, and to its perpetuation.

Attitude and behavior have always been twin aspects of the handicap of stuttering, and the role-expectations for clinicians vary accordingly. In the typical situation in which we are the sole clinician of the stutterer, we find ourselves wearing two hats. We are counselors or psychotherapists (in the broadest sense) with reference to the stutterer's feelings, and we are behavioral or speech clinicians with reference to his speaking pattern.

Some Principles of Counseling Stutterers

Let us concentrate on the attitudinal or feeling level, for it is here that the role of counseling enters most prominently. We may profit from emerging trends in counseling and psychotherapy generally, for we share the same presenting problems and challenges as do counselors and psychotherapists working with other designated problems.

A few specific principles of counseling the stutterer with emphasis on the feeling level, to relieve him of guilt associated with stuttering and other things, may be stated:

1. Create a relationship and an atmosphere in which he is able to express whatever he feels, without prior censorship. Help him understand that he is never wrong on the feeling level. In contrast, on the doing level, he has responsibility and choice.

2. Make the stutterer as a person the focus of therapy, not just the immediate suppression of stuttering frequency. Help him realize his potential for growth and development and self-realization.

3. Begin where the stutterer is, not where the clinician is. If he is fearful and overwhelmingly afraid to admit his fears, or feels guilty about them, give him running room enough to feel comfortable about what he feels.

4. Respect his feelings — guilt, shame, fear, or anger — as having an intrinsic validity, in terms of the kind of conditioning he has experienced in life.

5. Help him discover that the more guilt, shame and hatred he attaches to his stuttering, the more he will hold back, and the more he will be likely to stutter. Help him explore and share and diminish these loads of negative emotionality.

6. Deal with the **here** and **now**. Emphasize the possibilities of the future, not the mistakes of the past. "Where do we go from here? What behavior choices are available? What

can I do at this point?" Those are the questions that lead somewhere. Questions or statements like, "If only I hadn't done this," or "I wish this had happened differently," or "I am a failure," or "Why do things always go wrong for me?" tend to lead nowhere.

7. Let the stutterer know that you are interested in more than just his stuttering, that you are interested in him as a person. Get to know and understand him as a person as thoroughly as you can. He is better off if he feels you care about him and his feelings, that you are on his side whether he is a success or a failure in society's eyes, and that your emotional support doesn't have strings and conditions attached to it.

8. Be on the lookout for signs that he is trying to pretend more progress than he is actually experiencing, just to please you and retain your support.

9. As he reduces his load of shame, guilt, frustration and despair, help him prepare for the probability that progress and eventual recovery from the handicap of stuttering may still leave him with other problems with which he must cope. He may have to modify his view that stuttering has been the only impediment to his success; he may discover other problems, along with newly realized possibilities.

10. Beware of therapy-induced guilt, and at least be able to recognize it even if you can't entirely prevent some guilt development during the course of therapy. With a habit-based problem such as stuttering, it commonly happens that the stutterer finds, after coasting or wallowing in new-found fluency, he experiences an apparent return of the feelings and behaviors he thought he had conquered (Jost's Law of Habits). Unless continually practiced for a time, newly acquired responses drop out faster than older and more long-established response patterns. With relapse comes guilt — but the stutterer can be prepared for the possibility, and can reeestablish his improvement by the methods he used during therapy.

11. Every stutterer should be encouraged to develop initiative and independence of the therapist, and can learn in time to become his own clinical resource. The therapist can

help the stutterer shift from early dependence to later independence.

12. Fostering independence is not the same as abandonment, and the stutterer must always feel free to return to the clinician if new problems arise, or if he needs a refresher on dealing with the old ones.

13. Since some overlearning of newly acquired feelings and learned behavior patterns is desirable, the stutterer should not be dumped out of therapy the moment he becomes fluent, or more fluent than formerly. Stabilization for a considerable time after initial improvement is usually needed, to protect the gains made during the therapy, and to continue an abiding interest in the person and what he does with his life after improvement or recovery from the handicap of stuttering.